Clinical Management of Hypertension

5-20-04
Matthews
24.95

Seventh Edition

Marvin Moser, MD, FACP, FACC

Clinical Professor of Medicine,
Yale University School of Medicine

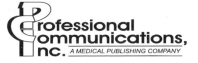

Professional Communications, Inc. *A MEDICAL PUBLISHING COMPANY*

Published by
Professional Communications, Inc.

Marketing Office:
400 Center Bay Drive
West Islip, NY 11795
(t) 631/661-2852
(f) 631/661-2167

Editorial Office:
PO Box 10
Caddo, OK 74729-0010
(t) 580/367-9838
(f) 580/367-9989

For orders only, please call
1-800-337-9838

or visit our website at
www.pcibooks.com

ISBN: 1-884735-92-4

Printed in the United States of America

DISCLAIMER
The opinions expressed in this publication reflect those of the author. However, the author makes no warranty regarding the contents of the publication. The protocols described herein are general and may not apply to a specific patient. Any product mentioned in this publication should be taken in accordance with the prescribing information provided by the manufacturer.

This text is printed on recycled paper.

DEDICATION

To the many hundreds of researchers and clinicians whose efforts have improved the management of hypertension and have helped to reduce morbidity and mortality from cardiovascular disease.

To the thousands of individuals involved in the National High Blood Pressure Education Program who have charted the course for better care of patients with hypertensive vascular disease.

And to the memory of Herbert Langford, Walter Kirkendall, Irvine Page, Harriet Dustan, and H. Michell Perry, colleagues and friends who helped define and clarify the hypertension "mosaic" and were active participants in the early efforts to manage hypertension.

ACKNOWLEDGMENT

I am indebted to Phyllis Freeny for her help in putting this manuscript into its final form;

To Adrienne Cramer, my research associate, for her help in all of our endeavors over the past 35-plus years; and

Finally, to the Hypertension Education Foundation, Inc. for research support.

TABLE OF CONTENTS

TABLES

FIGURES

About the Author

Dr. Moser is Clinical Professor of Medicine at the Yale University School of Medicine and was the senior medical advisor to the National High Blood Pressure Education Program of the National Heart, Lung and Blood Institute from 1974 to 2002. He was Chairman of the first Joint National Committee (JNC) on the Prevention, Detection, Evaluation, and Treatment of High Blood Pressure in 1977, Vice-Chairman of the committee in 1980, and has participated in each of the other five JNCs. Dr. Moser is Emeritus Chief of Cardiology, White Plains Hospital Medical Center, White Plains, New York. He is Editor in Chief of the *Journal of Clinical Hypertension* and the author of more than 400 scientific papers, 26 book chapters, and 11 books. These include *Myths, Misconceptions and Heroics, the Story of the Treatment of Hypertension*, published in 1997 and 2002, and *Clinical Management of Cardiovascular Risk Factors in Diabetes* (2002) (with James Sowers, MD).

He has received numerous awards for his contributions in the field of hypertension research and treatment.

Preface

This seventh edition of *Clinical Management of Hypertension* continues to update hypertension treatment recommendations with interpretations of new data. The most recent management guidelines of the Seventh Joint National Committee on Prevention, Detection, Evaluation, and Treatment of High Blood Pressure are critiqued. The 2003 European Society of Hypertension and Society of Cardiology guidelines and new treatment algorithm are also reviewed and evaluated. Recently introduced antihypertensive agents are discussed, and information from several long-term trials that have been completed within the past year is incorporated into treatment decisions.

Updates from several long-term trials, such as the Swedish Trial in Older Patients With Hypertension (STOP-Hypertension-2), the Nordic Diltiazem (NORDIL) trial, and the International Nifedipine Gastrointestinal Therapeutic System Study Intervention as a Goal for Hypertension Therapy (INSIGHT), will be discussed further and their results considered along with some of the more recent trials.

During the past year, several important long-term cardiovascular (CV)-event studies have been completed. The Antihypertensive and Lipid-Lowering Treatment to Prevent Heart Attack Trial (ALLHAT) was the first major comparison of a diuretic-based treatment program with a calcium channel blocker (CCB), an angiotensin-converting enzyme (ACE) inhibitor, and an α-blocker regimen. The results of this study have been questioned by some investigators and will be carefully reviewed. In addition, the Australian National Blood Pressure (ANBP 2) study has also been completed. This study compared a diuretic-based treatment program to an ACE inhibitor–based regimen and appeared to produce somewhat different results than ALLHAT; this, too, will be evaluated and put in perspective with regard to practical treatment considerations.

This seventh edition presents further comparisons of the older medications (diuretics and β-blockers) with newer therapies (ACE inhibitors and CCBs), especially as these relate to elderly patients. Many of the recent trials reveal new information about treating hypertension in older patients, especially those with systolic hypertension and diabetes. These will be reviewed in detail as the majority of patients with systolic hypertension are still not controlled at goal BP levels. Data on the treatment of the old and very old patient (>80 years of age) will be updated.

Numerous trials with angiotensin II receptor blockers (ARBs), especially in patients with diabetes and varying degrees of nephropathy, which were completed a year or two ago will be reviewed and put in perspective with the newer trials such as the Losartan Intervention for End-point Reduction in Hypertension (LIFE) trial. The implications of these studies for all hypertensives, including those patients with diabetes, are discussed. An update of findings from the Heart Outcomes Prevention Evaluation (HOPE) trial will also be discussed as they apply to current clinical practice.

In addition, newer trials evaluating the possible benefits of lowering blood pressure (BP) in patients after a stroke (ie, the PROGRESS trial) provide new insights into the treatment of this growing number of patients. The CONVINCE trial, comparing the use of standard therapy (diuretics/β-blockers) to that of a long-acting nondihydropyridine CCB, attempts to answer the question of whether chronotherapy is of value, ie, the use of medication at night with maximum effect during hours of arousal when more CV events occur. These major trials, data relating to a recently introduced aldosterone antagonist, as well as an update of the new definitions of hypertension and prehypertension, provide material that should be of interest to most clinicians.

This seventh edition again emphasizes the importance of utilizing the systolic blood pressure (SBP) as a major indicator of CV risk and guide to outcome. Failure to control SBP levels is probably the most important reason for poor BP control rates. Treatment to goal BPs—goals even lower than those previously recommended—represents a major challenge. The necessity to use multiple medications in addition to lifestyle interventions to achieve these goals will be reemphasized. Above all, this seventh edition of *Clinical Management of Hypertension* will send a clear message that:

- More individuals with hypertension should be treated
- Effective and safe treatment is available, and
- Achieving levels of BP as close to normal as possible—120-130/80-85 mm Hg—will reduce morbidity and mortality to an even greater degree than has occurred to date.

Appropriate treatment is available for most hypertensive patients but is not always being applied effectively.

Marvin Moser, MD
January 2004

1 Introduction

The management of hypertension has undergone a profound change since the 1940s and 1950s when many physicians were still not convinced that an elevated blood pressure (BP) increased the risk of cardiovascular (CV) disease. Treatment of hypertension was primitive and consisted of a rigid low-sodium diet that few people could follow, mutilative surgeries (such as sympathectomy or bilateral adrenalectomy), and a few medications whose toxic effects were deterrents to their widespread use. Studies in the late 1940s had established that if BP could be lowered in severe or malignant hypertension and sustained at lower levels, many cases of stroke and heart failure could be prevented and survival increased. Physicians began to treat patients with less severe hypertension in the 1960s to 1980s as data from several large clinical trials confirmed that even slight elevations of BP above an arbitrary limit of 140/90 mm Hg increased CV risk and that lowering BP that was above this level would decrease complications. As more information accumulated, it became apparent that the benefits of treating even less-severe degrees of hypertension far outweighed the risks, both in young and elderly subjects.

Clinical Management of Hypertension reviews these data and data from the more recent clinical trials as they apply to the practicing physician to provide guidance in making clinical decisions. It is not intended to be a complete textbook on hypertension and does not cover in-depth discussions of the diagnosis of secondary hypertension or specifics regarding the management of hypertension in children or in pregnancy; for that, the reader is referred to standard texts. It will, however, highlight recent advances in treatment and discuss a program that includes lifestyle interventions, including new data on the effects of sodium restriction and specific diets on BP as well as the use of older and newer medications.

The program outlined in this seventh edition represents our current approach to management, an approach that we have found to be practical and successful as it has evolved over the past 40-plus years. Not all medications within each class of drugs are discussed; choice of therapy is obviously an individual one, but specific suggestions have been made as to when and how we believe certain therapies should be used. Many of the data in the report of the Seventh Joint National Committee (JNC 7) on Prevention, Detection, Evaluation, and Treatment of High Blood Pressure, which was published in the *Journal of the American Medical Association* on May 21, 2003, as well as the 2003 recommendations of the European Society of Cardiology and European Society of Hypertension, are reviewed and critiqued.

In light of the results of the recent long-term trials, the recommendations of the JNC 7 for initial specific medical therapy will be reevaluated in this seventh edition of *Clinical Management of Hypertension*. Some of these recommendations, especially those suggesting the use of a thiazide diuretic as initial therapy in most patients and the designation of people with BPs between 120/80 and 139/89 mm Hg as "prehypertensives," have been criticized by some investigators. Reasons for these recommendations and criticisms will be reviewed. Much, but not all, of the material in the European guidelines is consistent with guidelines established by the JNC 7. The differences and similarities will be highlighted.

Specific details for the treatment of malignant or accelerated hypertension, hypertension in pregnancy, etc, can be found in the expanded version of JNC 7 and the European update and will not be reviewed.

We hope that this update of hypertension management will be of value to the primary care physician and internist in the treatment of hypertensive patients.

2 Diagnosis

As late as the 1960s, some physicians believed that an elevated blood pressure (BP) was necessary to provide an adequate blood supply to vital organs as people aged. Following the landmark Framingham Study and other epidemiologic studies (ie, Tecumseh, LA County), it became obvious, however, that as BP increases even from levels of 110-115/75-80 mm Hg, the risk for cardiovascular (CV) events increases. Risk increases more dramatically when BP rises to >140/90 mm Hg. Therefore, an arbitrary number was assigned as a definition of hypertension: ≥140/90 mm Hg. Later, it became apparent that lowering BP below this level decreases the incidence of CV events.

Classification of Hypertension

■ **Systolic Blood Pressure:**
   It Is Time to Change Our Emphasis
   For many years, it was also believed that diastolic blood pressure (DBP) was more important than systolic blood pressure (SBP) in defining future CV risk. More recent data, however, have established that elevated SBP may increase risk more than comparatively elevated DBP. For example, in the Multiple Risk Factor Intervention Trial (MRFIT), in which >300,000 men were tracked, SBP levels of 150-159 mm Hg conferred a greater relative risk for coronary heart disease (CHD) events than DBP levels of 95-100 mm Hg (**Figure 2.1**). Yet many physicians will treat patients with these levels of DBP and not intervene until SBP levels are considerably higher; recent data suggest that <25% of people with SBP >155-160 mm Hg are being treated.

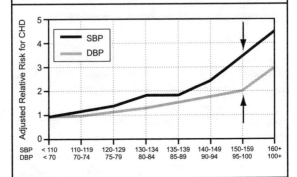

FIGURE 2.1 — RELATIVE RISK OF ELEVATED SYSTOLIC AND DIASTOLIC BLOOD PRESSURES

As noted, elevated systolic blood pressure (SBP) may impart greater risk for coronary heart disease (CHD) than diastolic blood pressure (DBP); ie, 150-159 mm Hg systolic blood pressure is greater risk than 95-100 mm Hg diastolic blood pressure. See text.

Data from: *JAMA*. 1990;263:1795-1801.

It has been clearly established that *isolated systolic hypertension* (ISH), still defined in some countries as SBP 160 mm Hg with DBP ≤90 mm Hg, also increases risk not only for stroke and congestive heart failure, but for CHD events as well. Of importance is the fact that lowering BP from these levels decreases morbidity and mortality. Recent data have also established that so-called isolated *borderline* systolic hypertension (ie, SBP 140-159 mm Hg with DBP <90 mm Hg) significantly increases risk for CV events and for the future development of more severe hypertension. A new definition of ISH includes SBP >140 mm Hg with DBP <90 mm Hg at any age and eliminates the designation of isolated borderline systolic hypertension. Approximately 60%-plus of persons >65 years of age have SBP >140 mm Hg. Patients with these levels of BP should initially be treated with lifestyle modifications. If SBP remains >145-150 mm Hg, medication may be tried. There is no proof as yet that morbidity or mortality is reduced by specific treatment in these patients with stage 1 ISH, but if BP can be lowered with a simple regimen without side effects, it is probably worthwhile.

The JNC 7 Blood Pressure Classification

The Seventh Joint National Committee (JNC 7) on Prevention, Detection, Evaluation, and Treatment of High Blood Pressure has redefined hypertension to conform to newer data defining risk (**Table 2.1**). Optimal BP in an adult is defined as <120/80 mm Hg.

The high-normal category of JNC 6 (BP 80-89/ 130-139 mm Hg) has been dropped. Instead, a new classification of "prehypertension" with BP between 120-130/80-89 mm Hg has been introduced (**Table 2.1**). This designation does not suggest that patients who have these BPs should be vigorously treated; rather, they should be followed and periodically re-evaluated because they are at greater risk for CV dis-

TABLE 2.1 — JNC 7 BLOOD PRESSURE CLASSIFICATION			
BP Classification	**SBP (mm Hg)**		**DBP (mm Hg)**
Normal	<120	and	<80
Prehypertension	120-139	or	80-89
Stage 1 hypertension	140-159	or	90-99
Stage 2 hypertension	≥160	or	≥100
Abbreviations: BP, blood pressure; DBP, diastolic blood pressure; SBP, systolic blood pressure.			
From: The JNC 7 Report. *JAMA*. 2003;289:2560-2572.			

ease than patients with lower BP, especially if they have other risk factors for heart disease (ie, diabetes, hyperlipidemia, or a history of smoking).

Numerous observers have questioned the designation and "labeling" of prehypertension in patients with BP levels between 120/80 and 139/89 mm Hg. The classification is based upon epidemiologic data that clearly indicate that risk gradually rises with an increasing level of SBP from 110 mm Hg (ie, risk is greater at 120 mm Hg than 110 mm Hg, greater at 130 mm Hg than 120 mm Hg, etc). The investigators who question the new recommendations argue that there are no data suggesting that reduction of BP from the number-defined prehypertension category is associated with benefit. Further, they postulate that the risk, although increased, does not appear to justify the labeling and treatment of a large number of people (perhaps as many as 20 million) as prehypertensive based upon available data. The question will probably have to be resolved by a long-term trial demonstrating that lowering BP from levels of prehypertension, not just in people with diabetes and/or kidney disease, but in all patients, is beneficial and reduces CV events. In the meantime, physicians should consider that people in the range of 130-140/80-90 mm Hg do have some increase in risk and all efforts to modify lifestyle should be followed. These measures are generally without risk and will reduce overall CV risk even if BP is not lowered significantly. However, overemphasis of the numbers is to be discouraged, especially in the absence of other recognized risk factors for CV disease.

The JNC 7 eliminated the stage 3 classification (≥180 mm Hg/≥110 mm Hg) that had appeared in previous reports. Severe hypertension is relatively rare and the approach to therapy is similar at BPs of 180-190/100 mm Hg or 210/120 mm Hg, except for patients with acute symptoms (ie, hypertensive urgencies or emergencies). The new classification is simpler and reflects additional data (**Table 2**.1)

The diagnosis of hypertension should not be based on one visit, unless BP is >160-165/100-105 mm Hg; specific treatment is clearly indicated in these instances. BP levels lower than these should be checked several times over a 3- to 6-month period (duration is dependent on the presence of other risk factors) as lifestyle modifications are made (see Chapter 3, *Lifestyle Modifications in the Management of Hypertension*). In our experience, BP returns toward normal levels in approximately 20% to 25% of subjects with stage 1 hypertension.

The European Cardiology and Hypertension Society guidelines classify hypertension as grades 1, 2, and 3 and continue to designate BP as optimal (<120/80 mm Hg), normal (120-129/80-84 mm Hg), and high-normal (130-139/85-89 mm Hg). This report encourages physicians to use risk factors other than the BP level to determine CV risk and urgency of treatment.

It is probably still appropriate to define hypertension as BP >140/90 mm Hg based on epidemiologic evidence and data that CV events are decreased in persons whose BP is lowered to <140/90 mm Hg.

■ **Pulse Pressure**: **Should This Be the Criterion of Risk**?

There has been a recent emphasis on the importance of elevated pulse pressures, ie, pulse pressure of >60 or 65 mm Hg. For example, BP levels of 150-160/90 mm Hg with a pulse pressure of 60-70 confers a greater risk of CV disease than a BP of 135-145/95 mm Hg with a pulse pressure of 40-50, despite the higher DBP.

An increased pulse pressure correlates fairly closely with aging and less-elastic large arteries. Currently, however, using SBP as a measure of risk and a determinant of treatment appears to be reasonable and less complicated than changing the approach to management based on levels of pulse pressure. Recent studies have reaffirmed that SBP is an accurate predictor of outcome.

The rush to embrace SBP as the risk marker has led some physicians to forget about the importance of an elevated DBP. This is unfortunate; elevated DBP (>90 mm Hg) remains a good prognostic indicator, especially in young and middle-aged individuals. DBP levels tend to decrease (as SBP increases) in people >55 years of age.

It is of interest to note that about 90% of cases would be classified correctly for possible antihypertensive drug therapy if only SBP was used as a criterion. About 20% would be correctly classified as hypertensive if only the DBP was used.

"White-Coat" Hypertension

Approximately 20% of people experience BP that is higher in a doctor's office than at home. These patients should not be ignored. They may already have physiologic changes when compared with people whose BP is normal at home *and* in a doctor's office:

- Vascular resistance tends to be increased.
- There may be evidence of left ventricular diastolic dysfunction.
- Chemically, they resemble patients with early hypertension, ie, there is evidence of increased insulin resistance, and lipid levels tend to be higher.
- More patients with "white-coat" hypertension are obese and have diabetes than those who are normotensive (in office and at home).

The question arises, should patients be screened for white-coat or "office" hypertension and undergo ambulatory BP monitoring or should decisions regarding treatment be made on the basis of office readings or home BP recordings?

Based on available data and our own experience, we believe that office BPs are reliable indicators of outcome. If BP is not reduced to normal levels (<140/ 90 mm Hg) during the 3- to 6-month period of observation and lifestyle interventions, the patient should be treated with medication, regardless of the level of home or work-site pressures. This may appear to be an aggressive approach to management but is consistent with extensive data.

Ambulatory Blood Pressure Monitoring: Is This Procedure Necessary to Establish a Diagnosis?

It should be pointed out that all of the data upon which we base our estimates of risk were accumulated from casual BP readings taken in an office or clinic. The higher the casual BP, the greater the risk of a CV event. It should also be remembered that the data upon which we estimate benefit of treatment are also based on casual BPs. In clinical trials, such as the Systolic Hypertension in the Elderly Program (SHEP), the Hypertension Detection and Follow-up Program (HDFP), and the Antihypertensive and Lipid-Lowering Treatment to Prevent Heart Attack Trial (ALLHAT), BP was taken in an office or clinic every 3 to 4 months; patients with the lowest BP had the best outcome.

Ambulatory BP monitoring has contributed important information on the circadian rhythm of BP, establishing that BP decreases during sleeping hours and increases within an hour or two of arousal in the morning. It has helped to define a certain subset of patients whose BPs do not decrease from 2 AM to 6 AM. These so-called "nondippers" are more likely to have left ventricular hypertrophy (LVH). This phenomenon is more common in the black population.

There are also data suggesting that 24-hour BPs correlate more closely than office BPs with target-organ involvement. But whether or not LVH is present, some therapy should be instituted if casual BPs are consistently >140/90 mm Hg. Although ambulatory monitoring has proved to be an interesting research tool and is useful in establishing the duration of action of new drugs, it has not been recommended by any of the JNCs, including JNC 7, as a *routine* procedure in the initial evaluation of the hypertensive patient. We agree with this recommendation and do not believe that the use of this procedure is justified at this time. Nor do we believe that the data provided influence therapeutic decisions in a majority of patients.

Some patients want to know their BP. In these cases, or in situations where symptoms are confusing (eg, dizziness—is this the result of BP that is too high or too low?), BP can be taken at home with an inexpensive sphygmomanometer. A series of readings over time at different times of the day may actually provide more information than one 24-hour recording. A recent analysis of available electronic BP machines concluded that most of these are as accurate as aneroid instruments. They are relatively inexpensive and easy to use without the need for a stethoscope. Currently, the use of finger BP recorders cannot be recommended, although these are being improved and standardized.

Diagnostic Evaluation

As have all previous JNCs, the JNC 7 suggested a relatively inexpensive and simple diagnostic evaluation. This includes a careful history, physical examination, electrocardiogram (ECG), urinalysis, and blood chemistries that help to rule out not only renal failure (based on serum creatinine levels) but also a possible secondary cause of hypertension (eg, primary aldosteronism) by checking serum potassium levels. A lipid profile and blood glucose levels are also suggested to help identify other CV risk factors (**Table 2.2**). These recommendations have not changed significantly since the first JNC report in 1977.

TABLE 2.2 — SUGGESTED INITIAL EVALUATION OF THE PATIENT WITH HYPERTENSION

- History and physical examination
- Urinalysis
- Chemical profile, including creatinine, blood glucose, potassium, uric acid, and lipids
- Electrocardiogram
- Renin, catecholamines and aldosterone levels are NOT recommended in the initial evaluation unless there are specific clinical clues to indicate the need

Data from: The JNC 7 Report. *JAMA*. 2003;289:2560-2572.

An Echocardiogram—Should It Be Done as a Routine Procedure?

An ECG was suggested by all of the JNCs to detect arrhythmias and evidence of ischemic heart disease. An echocardiogram has not been recommended as a *routine* procedure for the following reason: It is recognized that an echocardiogram is a more sensitive indicator of LVH than an ECG. However, as noted, patients whose BPs remain >140/90 mm Hg after several recordings and several months of lifestyle intervention should have their BP lowered with medication, regardless of whether LVH is present. In addition, although some investigators believed for many years that the presence or absence of LVH should be used as a guide for specific initial therapy, it has now been demonstrated in several recent studies that all of the drugs that are *currently used as monotherapy or in combination*, ie, diuretics, β-blockers, angiotensin-converting enzyme (ACE) inhibitors, angiotensin II receptor blockers (ARBs), or calcium channel blockers, will reverse LVH if BP is lowered. ACE inhibitors (and possibly ARBs) and diuretics are probably more effective than the other agents. It is therefore unnecessary to order an echocardiogram in the initial evaluation of the hypertensive patient unless there is another specific indication for this procedure.

Additional studies over and above those recommended in **Table 2.2** may be necessary in:

- Patients with hypertension who are <15 years of age
- Elderly patients (>65 years of age) with recent onset of moderately severe or severe hypertension
- Individuals with persistent elevations of BP after triple-drug therapy that includes a diuretic
- People with hypertension and symptoms of headache or unusual patterns of sweating and palpitations.

In these instances, procedures to rule out renovascular disease, primary aldosteronism, or pheochromocytoma should be undertaken. Details of these procedures can be found in any standard textbook on hypertension.

Summary

Hypertensive patients should be approached with a confident attitude that the complications that used to occur in many patients can be prevented. The diagnostic evaluation is relatively simple in the majority of cases and does not routinely require an echocardiogram or ambulatory BP monitoring. In most cases, office BPs should be used to estimate risk and judge prognosis. More attention should be paid to elevated SBP than has been in the past. This measurement has been found to be a better predictor of risk than DBP and has often been ignored in making treatment decisions. Some form of treatment should be undertaken in anyone whose BP remains >140/90 mm Hg after repeated observations.

3

Lifestyle Modifications in the Management of Hypertension

If blood pressure (BP) is >140/90 mm Hg but <160/100 mm Hg during an initial examination, a definite diagnosis of hypertension is not justified, but some form of intervention is indicated. Several BP readings should be taken and the numbers averaged. Nonpharmacologic or lifestyle modifications should be suggested and another visit scheduled for an additional BP check and confirmation of the diagnosis. If, however, BP is >160-165/100-105 mm Hg on the initial visit, specific medical therapy plus lifestyle modifications are probably indicated, even in the absence of other cardiovascular (CV) risk factors.

There are numerous lifestyle modifications advocated for lowering BP. Many of them, however, may not be effective. Although everyone would like to be in charge of their own destiny and manage a disease process without the use of medication or other treatments, this is often not possible in the management of hypertension. A list of possible lifestyle changes is shown in **Table 3.1**.

Weight Loss

A high percentage of people with elevated BP are obese. It is well known that obesity predisposes people to hypertension and diabetes. Upper-body or abdominal obesity (more common in men), so-called android or apple-shaped obesity, is more frequently associated with dyslipidemia, diabetes, and elevated BP than obesity involving the buttocks or thighs. The latter is more common in women, and is called gynecoid or pear-

**TABLE 3.1 — LIFESTYLE MODIFICATIONS
FOR CONTROL OF HYPERTENSION AND/OR
OVERALL CARDIOVASCULAR RISK**

- Weight loss, if overweight*
- Reduction of sodium intake to less than 100 mmol/day (2.4 g of sodium or approximately 6 g of sodium chloride)*
- Limit alcohol intake to <1 oz/day of ethanol (24 oz of beer, 10 oz of wine, or 2 oz of 80-proof whiskey); approximately one half of these amounts for women and thin people
- Cessation of smoking and reduction of dietary saturated fat and cholesterol for overall cardio-vascular health; reduced fat intake also helps reduce caloric intake—important for control of weight and type 2 diabetes
- Maintain adequate dietary potassium, calcium, and magnesium intake
- Relaxation techniques—biofeedback
- Vegetarian diets, fish oil

* These interventions have been found to be most effective. Data on other interventions are not definitive (see text).

Modified from: The JNC 7 Report. *JAMA*. 2003;289:2560-2572.

shaped obesity. The most effective method to possibly *prevent* the development of hypertension in normotensive individuals or to possibly lower BP in hypertensive individuals is to maintain normal weight or, if obese, to lose weight. Many patients do not know what their ideal weight should be. **Table 3.2** describes how to estimate ideal weight. This is a useful guide for discussions with patients.

People who exceed these limits by 20% or more are considered obese and should be started on a weight-reduction program. Experience shows that liq-

TABLE 3.2 — HOW TO ESTIMATE **IDEAL BODY WEIGHT***	
Women — Height: 5 feet, 5 inches	
Allow 100 pounds for first 5 feet of height	100
Add 5 pounds for each additional inch	+ 25
Ideal body weight for a 5-foot, 5-inch woman = 125	
Men — Height: 5 feet, 10 inches	
Allow 106 pounds for first 5 feet of height	106
Add 6 pounds for each additional inch	+ 60
Ideal body weight for a 5-foot, 10-inch man = 166	
* A variation of between 5 and 10 lbs is probably acceptable.	

uid formulas, "crash," or "miracle" diets are ineffective over the long term. The process of losing large amounts of weight quickly leads to a downward readjustment of the metabolic rate and a gain in weight once a more normal diet is resumed. A simple, easy-to-follow weight-reduction program, resulting in a loss of one or two pounds per week, is most effective. In cases of morbid obesity (ie, 100% or more above ideal weight), more stringent methods should be undertaken.

There is currently a wave of enthusiasm for a high-fat, high-protein, low-carbohydrate intake to lose weight. There is little doubt that weight loss occurs; the resulting ketosis decreases appetite and total calorie intake is reduced. The total intake of calories does count! But the abundant data regarding the long-term CV risk of a high-fat intake cannot be ignored. Until there are better long-term safety data for these diets, they should not be encouraged. A balanced intake, such as the Dietary Approaches to Stop Hypertension (DASH) diet, makes more sense.

Table 3.3 illustrates how to calculate the number of calories necessary to *maintain* ideal weight. This can serve as a starting point in calculating behavioral and dietary changes. In a person who usually ingests about 2,000 calories a day and is targeted to lose one pound a week, daily caloric intake should be reduced by 500 calories or, as an alternative, reduced by 300 calories and caloric expenditure (exercise) increased by about 200 calories a day. An overall reduction of about 500 calories a day from the usual intake will result in a weight loss of approximately one pound a week (3,500 calories equal one pound). **Table 3.4** summarizes the caloric expenditures for various activities.

Weight loss is difficult to accomplish, but if achieved and maintained, it will usually result in some decrease in BP. This may be enough in some patients

---

TABLE 3.3 — HOW TO ESTIMATE NUMBER OF CALORIES NEEDED TO MAINTAIN IDEAL BODY WEIGHT

Multiply ideal weight (not necessarily present weight) by activity level. Example:

Ideal weight (lbs)	125
Activity level*	× 13*
Total calories needed per day to maintain ideal weight	= 1,625

A sedentary woman whose ideal weight is 125 will require approximately 125 × 13 or 1,625 calories/day to maintain her ideal weight. More than this will result in a weight gain.

* Sedentary activity level is used for example. Use 15 and 17 for moderately active and very active activity levels, respectively.

TABLE 3.4 — CALORIE EXPENDITURES FOR VARIOUS ACTIVITIES

Activity	Approximate # of calories burned per *half-hour*
Normal Activities	
Cleaning windows	130
Gardening	110
Mowing lawn (power mower)	125
Sitting/conversing	40
Vacuuming	130
Moderate Exercise	
Bicycling (5 mph)	105
Bicycling (8 mph)	165
Bowling	135
Playing golf (using power cart)	100
Playing golf (pulling cart)	135
Playing volleyball	175
Roller skating	175
Swimming (1/4 mph)	150
Walking (1 mph)	65
Walking (3 mph)	140
Vigorous Exercise	
Bicycling (10 mph)	195
Bicycling (13 mph)	330
Hill climbing (100 ft/hr)	245
Ice skating (10 mph)	200
Jogging (5 mph)	265
Playing squash, handball	300
Playing tennis	210
Running (8 mph)	360
Skiing (10 mph)	300
Walking (4 mph)	195

3

with slightly elevated BP (stage 1) to reduce their BP to normotensive levels (<140/90 mm Hg). There is no risk and this intervention need not be costly if it is carried out without involvement in health clubs or expensive "miracle weight-loss" programs. Weight loss is particularly beneficial in diabetic patients or those with hyperlipidemia. It has been estimated from study data that a loss of about 20 pounds will result in a decrease of SBP of about 5 to 20 mm Hg (**Table 3.5**).

TABLE 3.5 — LIFESTYLE MODIFICATIONS	
	Approximate SBP Reduction (Range/mm Hg)
Weight reduction	5-20/10 kg of weight loss
DASH eating plan	8-14
Dietary sodium reduction	2-8
Physical activity	4-9
Moderation of alcohol consumption	2-4
Abbreviations: DASH, Dietary Approaches to Stop Hypertension; SBP, systolic blood pressure.	

Attempts at weight loss (if appropriate) should be begun and the patient seen again in 2 to 3 months for a repeat BP check. If the BP is now <140/90 mm Hg in the person whose BP was initially >140/90 mm Hg but <160/100 mm Hg, weight loss (if accomplished) may have been a factor in reducing BP, but BP may have come down anyway (if the patient had initial BP >160/100 mm Hg, he/she would probably have been taking medication). In all of the large hypertension clinical trials, a varying percentage of about 10% to 15% of people experienced a decrease in BP without specific interventions. As noted, in addition to its immediate effect on BP, achieving normal weight may be important in preventing diabetes or future hypertension. If, however, BP remains elevated and specific therapy becomes necessary, maintaining an ideal weight will be helpful in minimizing the amount of medication. Recent studies in the elderly indicate a decrease in the need for medication in about 30% of patients who achieve a weight loss of about 8 to 10 pounds with or without sodium restriction. Weight reduction of even 10 or 15 pounds (even without specific sodium restriction) will also lower BP in some younger and middle-aged patients.

Sodium Restriction

Epidemiologic and animal data have established a clear link between sodium intake and elevated BP. Yet, conflicting reports have confused physicians about the importance of sodium reduction in the treatment of hypertension. Most people ingest more salt (sodium) than needed. The average salt intake in the United States is still approximately 10 g/day (approximately 4 g/day sodium). Little harm would be done if every person reduced sodium intake. In a patient with even transiently elevated BP, the reduction of salt intake to approximately 6 g/day (sodium to approximately 2.4 g or about 100 mmol/day) may result in a decrease of about 2 to 8 mm Hg in SBP. The benefits of sodium moderation may be especially evident in the elderly and in black patients who are usually more "salt sensitive" than other people.

Some studies report significant decreases in BP with moderate sodium restriction; others report only insignificant changes. Many of these trials, however, have been poorly controlled or are short term and include few subjects. Recent data from the well-controlled randomized Trial of Nonpharmacologic Interventions in the Elderly (TONE) study indicate that a reduction of about 30% to 40% in daily sodium intake (with or without weight loss) resulted in a lowering of BP and a decrease in the amount of medication required to maintain normotensive BP levels.

The recently completed DASH low-sodium study was a carefully controlled trial that evaluated the BP lowering effects of progressively lower-sodium diets with all other nutrients kept constant. In this trial, some BP decrease was noted in those hypertensive subjects on a diet of approximately 2.5-g/day sodium intake compared with those on a relatively high-sodium diet that included approximately 3 g/day sodium. A further clinically significant BP decrease was noted in patients on a diet containing about 1.5 g/day sodium compared with those on diets containing 2.5 and 3.0+ g/day. BP decreases were also noted in normotensive individuals who reduced their sodium intake. A greater BP response was noted in black subjects. Although this was a "feeding" trial, with all foods provided to the subjects, and may not be applicable to the real world, the results indicate what might be accomplished by sodium restriction to levels lower than currently advised.

Currently, there is no positive way to identify a person whose BP would be lowered by sodium restriction (salt-sensitive individuals). But sodium restriction to the degree possible in clinical practice is not harmful and therefore should be a part of the treatment regimen for the hypertensive patient. This approach is also reasonable in persons who may be normotensive but have a family history of hypertension.

Table 3.6 lists some foods with a high sodium content. If these are avoided or markedly restricted, many patients can reduce their sodium intake to a reasonable level and possibly lower BP without further, more difficult-to-follow restrictions. More rigid salt restriction is necessary for patients with renal failure or congestive heart failure. Sodium restriction (1 to 1.5 g sodium or <75 mmol/day) might also be

TABLE 3.6 — SOME FOODS WITH A HIGH SODIUM CONTENT THAT SHOULD BE AVOIDED

- Potato chips
- Pretzels
- Salted crackers
- Biscuits
- Pancakes
- Fast foods
- Olives
- Pickles
- Sauerkraut
- Soy sauce
- Catsup
- Many kinds of cheese
- Commercially prepared soups or stews
- Pastries or cakes made from self-rising flour mixes
- Bouillon
- Ham
- Sausages
- Frankfurters
- Smoked meats or fish
- Sardines
- Tomato juice (canned)
- Frozen lima beans
- Frozen peas
- Canned spinach
- Canned carrots

effcctive in lowering BP to a greater degree in other patients as noted in the DASH trial. Most people find it impossible, however, to follow this type of regimen for other than short periods, and it may not be necessary.

A study suggesting that marked sodium restriction might actually increase the occurrence of myocardial infarction was poorly designed and has not been confirmed. Results from this study should not be used for treatment decisions.

Moderate salt restriction should be tried in all individuals with elevated BP. The so-called salt-sensitive subject may experience a definite decrease in BP within a few days or weeks. In others, there may be no response at all. As noted, this individual variation in response cannot be accurately predicted. From a public health point of view, *moderation of sodium intake and weight loss or maintaining normal weight have proven to be the most effective methods for preventing hypertension.*

Calcium Supplementation

Data are confusing concerning the value of calcium supplementation. Some investigators maintain the following:

- A low calcium intake predisposes patients to hypertension
- An increase in calcium intake with 1 g to 2 g of supplemental calcium lowers BP.

Others interpret the available information differently. Based on current data, calcium supplements cannot be recommended as effective, definitive treatment for hypertension. In postmenopausal women, supplemental calcium is probably useful in the prevention and treatment of osteoporosis. An adequate calcium intake as in the DASH diet is suggested for all hypertensive individuals.

Potassium Supplementation

A high potassium intake prevents stroke in animal models and some recent epidemiologic data suggest a reduction in humans as well. Supplements of 60 to 100 mEq/day above the usual dietary intake of between 50 and 80 mEq/day have been shown to lower BP in humans in some clinical trials. Some patients will develop gastrointestinal symptoms with this degree of potassium supplementation. A dietary potassium intake of about 60 to 100 mEq/day is recommended regardless of whether hypertension is present. In areas like the rural South where the daily intake of potassium may be low (<40 mEq/day) and daily intake of sodium high (>5 g/day), there is a high prevalence of hypertension and stroke. Some investigators strongly believe that the ratio of sodium to potassium intake is a more important predictor of elevated BP than the intake of either of those minerals alone, ie, less sodium and more potassium is advocated. At present, however, there is little evidence to support the use of *potassium supplements* as *definitive therapy* for hypertension. **Table 3.7** lists some foods that are high in potassium. A diet high in fruits and vegetables (similar to the DASH diet) will provide an adequate potassium intake.

For many years, attempts have been made to reduce sodium and increase potassium intake by the use of potassium salt substitutes. Many of these substitutes are bitter to the taste and poorly tolerated. In some patients on thiazide diuretics, potassium (as well as magnesium) supplementation may be necessary. The use of potassium-sparing diuretics will help prevent both potassium and magnesium deficiencies.

Magnesium Supplementation

There is some evidence from animal studies that a high magnesium intake lowers BP. Other data suggest that an increase in magnesium intake may lower BP in hypertensive individuals and may reduce the incidence of stroke. Currently, magnesium supplements cannot be recommended as a definitive method for lowering BP, but all of the recent Joint National Committees (JNCs) on Prevention, Detection, Evaluation, and Treatment of High Blood Pressure have appropriately recommended that an adequate intake of this mineral, as well as potassium, be maintained. A well-balanced diet that includes fruits and vegetables will usually supply adequate amounts of magnesium.

High-Fiber, Low-Fat Diet; Fish Oil; Garlic

High-fiber, low-fat diets have also been shown to reduce BP in some studies, but carefully controlled long-

TABLE 3.7 — LOW-SALT, HIGH-POTASSIUM FOODS

Food	Serving Size	Potassium* (mg)	Sodium† (mg)
Apricots	3 medium	281	1
Apricots (dried)	8 halves	490	13
Asparagus	6 spears	278	2
Avocado	1/2 medium	604	4
Banana	1 medium	569	1
Beans (white, cooked)	1/2 cup	416	7
Beans (green)	1 cup	189	5
Broccoli	1 stalk	267	10
Cantaloupe	1/4 medium	251	12
Carrots	2 small	341	47
Dates	10 medium	648	1
Grapefruit	1/2 medium	135	1
Mushrooms	4 large	414	15
Orange	1 medium	311	2
Orange juice	1 cup	496	3
Peach	1 medium	202	1
Peanuts (plain)	2 1/2 oz	740	2
Potato	1 medium	504	4
Prunes (dried)	8 large	940	11
Raisins	1/4 medium	271	10
Spinach	1/2 cup	291	45
Squash (acorn)	1/2 baked	749	2
Sunflower seeds	3 1/2 oz	920	30
Sweet potato	1 small	367	15
Tomato	1 small	244	3
Watermelon	1 slice (6 1/2 in)	600	6

* 1000 mg = 25.6 mmols.
† 1000 mg = 44 mmols.

term studies have not been done. Currently, there is little definitive evidence that this type of dietary intervention will lower BP. It may, however, be effective in maintaining serum lipid levels at more desirable levels. A low-fat, high-fiber diet can therefore be recommended.

Large doses of omega-3 fatty acids may lower BP to some extent but may produce adverse reactions. A meta-analysis that included results of this type of intervention from six trials in hypertensive patients reported a BP decrease of –5.5/–3.5 mm Hg. Dosages used were 6 to 10 capsules a day of commercially available fish oil, which is equivalent to a daily serving of 200 g of fish with a high content of omega-3 oils (eg, mackerel, certain kinds of salmon). This approach also cannot be recommended at this time as specific treatment for hypertension.

There is no good evidence that an extra daily intake of garlic will lower BP.

A diet rich in vegetables, fruits, and low-fat dairy products with reduced saturated and total fat (ie, the DASH diet) has been shown to reduce BP in individuals with either normal BP or with BP >140/90 mm Hg. BP reduction in hypertensive individuals and those with normal BPs were –11.4/–5.5 and –3.5/–2.4 mm Hg, respectively. This type of diet may possibly prevent the development of hypertension in some people. As noted in the original DASH diet study, sodium intake was not reduced, but a follow-up study with varying degrees of sodium restriction indicated that this is an additional effective method of lowering BP. To reiterate, the DASH diet was a diet in which all food was supplied to the study participants; results may not be relevant to clinical practice, but suggest what might be accomplished.

Alcohol Moderation

The JNC 7 recommended what the previous committees had suggested and numerous epidemiologic studies have reported. A low-to-moderate intake of alcohol may actually decrease CV risk, but an intake greater than about 2 oz/day ethanol may increase BP. Daily intake should not exceed 2 ounces of 80-proof whiskey, 10 ounces of wine, or 24 ounces of beer. Women and thin individuals should limit their ethanol intake to approximately one half of these amounts. We have followed patients who have been diagnosed as hypertensive whose BP has decreased to normal when alcohol intake was reduced from more than four to five drinks per day to one or none. A 2-year, carefully controlled study in >600 men evaluated the possibility of BP control by reducing alcohol intake and concluded that BP reduction is modest; however, the reduction in alcohol consumption in this trial was not as great as the investigators had anticipated. This approach cannot be considered definitive treatment. Alcohol probably contributes to elevated BP by its stimulatory effect on catecholamines. *The recommendation for a moderate intake of alcohol should obviously not be given to those with a strong family history of alcoholism or a personal sensitivity to alcohol.*

Exercise

Exercise is another confusing issue. Several studies have found that vigorous exercise over the short term will lower BP in patients with stage 1 or less severe hypertension, ie, between 140/90 and 160/100 mm Hg. Many of these studies were poorly controlled; in the studies that have had a control group, the difference between treated and control groups has usually not been great. On the other hand, the chance of a sedentary individual developing hypertension or a coronary event is greater than that of a physically active individual; this has been repeatedly demonstrated in long-term, prospective, epidemiologic studies.

There is some confusion over what constitutes an active person. Active does not imply involvement in vigorous aerobic exercises to achieve ≥75% or more of target heart rates that have been recommended by many exercise physiologists.

Recent data show that *CV risk* can be reduced by a program involving moderate exercise. This includes walking for 30 to 40 minutes three to four times per week at a rate of 2 to 3 miles per hour. Achieving *fitness* does require more vigorous aerobic activity, but someone can be an *active* individual without being *fit*, and a high level of fitness does not have to be achieved to reduce CV risk. Exercise is helpful in burning calories, thereby helping to reduce weight. Exercise may also increase vasodilator hormones that lower vascular resistance and may therefore help to lower BP. A program of brisk walking (30 minutes most days of the week) may reduce systolic blood pressure (SBP) by about 4-9 mm Hg. Exercise is recommended but is not to be counted on as definitive antihypertensive therapy.

Relaxation Programs and Biofeedback

Numerous relaxation and biofeedback programs have been advocated for the lowering of BP. These include yoga, transcendental meditation, and hypnosis. Most reported studies are poorly controlled. BP may be lowered at the time someone is practicing a relaxation technique, but this should not be depended on as definitive treatment. **Table 3.8** outlines the Benson technique for relaxation. Patients can be taught to do

TABLE 3.8 — DR. HERBERT BENSON'S RELAXATION RESPONSE TECHNIQUE

- Sit quietly in a comfortable position.
- Close your eyes.
- Relax all your muscles, progressing from your feet to your face. Keep them relaxed.
- Breathe through your nose. As you breathe out, say the word "one" silently to yourself.
- Continue for 10 to 20 minutes. You may open your eyes to check the time, but do not set an alarm. When you finish, sit quietly for several minutes, at first with your eyes closed. Do not stand for a few minutes.
- Do not worry about achieving a deep level of relaxation. Maintain a passive attitude and permit relaxation to occur at its own pace. When distracting thoughts occur, don't dwell upon them, but return to repeating "one." With practice, the response should come with little effort. Use the technique once or twice daily, but not within 2 hours after any meal, because the digestive processes seem to interfere with elicitation of the response.

To utilize this technique once or twice a day requires an ongoing commitment of time and effort.

Adapted from: *The Relaxation Response*. New York, NY: Times Books; 1984.

this in a few minutes. Using this technique once or twice a day cannot hurt anyone and may periodically reduce catecholamine levels and lower BP. Many of our patients have found this type of relaxation to be helpful without a major time or economic commitment.

Summary of Lifestyle Changes

After the initial discovery of elevated BP, the patient should be advised to:

- Reduce excess body weight by calorie restriction, if appropriate.
- Reduce dietary sodium to ≤6 g/day sodium chloride (≤2.4 g sodium).
- Maintain an adequate intake of potassium, calcium, and magnesium without necessarily using supplements (fruits, vegetables, and less-fat diary products).
- Limit alcohol intake to less than 2 oz of 80-proof whiskey, 10 oz of wine, or 24 oz of beer a day (approximately one half of these amounts for women and thin individuals).
- Exercise moderately within the framework of daily activity for 30 to 40 minutes, three to four times a week.
- Plan some type of relaxation for short periods several times a day.

In addition, because smoking and elevated lipid levels are important risk factors for heart disease, these should be corrected if present. There is no evidence that chronic smoking will cause a persistent elevation of BP, but smoking may have an immediate effect and raise BP, primarily because of the nicotine effect on catecholamines. If someone smokes ≥20 cigarettes per day, the recurrent elevations of BP may be harmful.

The Effects of Coffee on Blood Pressure

Should people with hypertension drink coffee that contains caffeine? Although some studies have reported that coffee intake can elevate BP more in hypertensive patients or those with "high normal BP" than in normotensive individuals, most of these studies have included the ingestion of more than four to five cups a day, or the equivalent amount of caffeine in several cups at one time. Although caffeine may elevate BP to some extent, presumably by its effect on sympathetic nerve activity, there appears to be no reason why people with hypertension cannot enjoy one to three cups of filtered coffee a day (but not usually at the same time). Some patients who monitor their BP at home might wish to check it before and about 30 minutes after a cup of coffee to judge the effect of the coffee. If a rise in SBP of >10-15 mm Hg occurs, it might be prudent to monitor this effect more closely.

If elevated BPs persist for more than an hour or two after a cup of coffee, then the use of decaffeinated coffee is indicated. Recent data suggest that the ingestion of an amount of caffeine equivalent to two to three cups of coffee (consumed at one time) may have unfavorable effects on blood vessel function. Caffeine-containing soft drinks and strong tea may also increase BP levels, but the clinical significance of these changes has not been defined.

Follow-Up Program

Although it may seem inappropriate to undertake *any* kind of intervention after only one BP reading, the above rather simple nonpharmacologic interventions:
- Make good sense
- Do no harm
- Incur no cost
- Require very little time on the part of the patient.

Even if the interventions have no effect on BP, they establish a pattern of behavior that can help to reduce the risk of heart disease.

Patients should be seen after 3 to 4 months if initial BP ranges between 140-150/90-95 mm Hg and sooner if BP levels are higher. If BP is still elevated >140/90 mm Hg despite lifestyle interventions but is not >150/95 mm Hg and no other risk factors are present, some experts believe that an additional 3-month trial of nonpharmacologic intervention may be justified (although specific therapy is clearly indicated if other major risk factors, such as smoking, diabetes, or hyperlipidemia, are present). I personally believe that specific drug therapy is the preferred approach at this stage, even if there are *no other* risk factors (see Chapter 4, *Drug Treatment of Hypertension: General Information*). If the BP is >150/95-100 mm Hg, specific medical therapy should certainly be undertaken regardless of whether other risk factors are present. On a third visit (2 to 3 months later) in subjects not already on medication, medical therapy is indicated if BPs are >140/90 mm Hg. This is true regardless of whether left ventricular hypertrophy or any other target-organ damage has been identified.

The 1999 World Health Organization–International Society of Hypertension (WHO-ISH) report recommends continuing monitoring without drug therapy even after 1 year of follow-up in patients with BP between 140/90 and 150/95 mm Hg without other risk factors. The recent European guidelines in 2003 also suggest long-term monitoring (up to 1 year) in patients at low risk (without other risk factors). If BP remains between 140-159/90-99 mm Hg after 3 to 12 months, drug treatment should be considered.

This approach is hard to justify and appears to ignore treatment and epidemiologic data. For example, there is evidence that pharmacologic intervention in addition to lifestyle modifications at this BP level will provide beneficial effects and reduce CV risk. This was demonstrated in a study of stage 1 hypertension (Treatment of Mild Hypertension Study [TOMHS]); a reduction in overall CV events was noted after 4 years in patients treated with antihypertensive drugs plus lifestyle interventions compared with those who were just continued on lifestyle interventions (average pretreatment BP was 140/91 mm Hg).

The European guidelines, however, are very specific regarding the treatment of elevated BP in the face of one or more other risk factors. For example, a patient is classified as very high risk if there is any evidence of clinical coronary heart disease. In those cases, even patients with SBP 135-139 mm Hg or DBP 85-89 mm Hg should probably be placed on drug therapy. In addition, patients with grade 1 or grade 2 (stage 1 or stage 2) hypertension with diabetes, any evidence of target organ involvement, or associated coronary heart disease should also be started on drug therapy without a specific evaluation of BP over a period of several months. In patients at moderate risk, however, the European recommendations suggest a trial of non-pharmacologic therapy for approximately 3 months and drug treatment instituted if BP remains DBP >140 mm Hg or SBP >90 mm Hg. As noted, we believe that even patients at low risk (without other risk factors), not just patients at moderate risk, should be treated with medication after this period of time on nonpharmacologic intervention.

Many patients have been led to believe that nonpharmacologic or lifestyle interventions are all that is necessary to control their BP—just lose weight, reduce salt intake, and exercise more. This is not true in most cases. This message has been repeated frequently and widely disseminated by the media and may represent a disservice to many people with hypertension. The exact numbers are not known, but our experience suggests that BP will be reduced to normal in <20% to 25% of all patients who have consistently elevated BP and who follow the above program. This is important to remember but it is also important to realize that long-term outcome may be adversely affected if lifestyle modifications are continued without medication, despite persistently elevated BP.

4

Drug Treatment of Hypertension: General Information

As noted in Chapter 3, *Lifestyle Modifications in the Management of Hypertension*, opinions differ as to when medication should be started. Patients with blood pressure (BP) in the range of about 140-150/90-100 mm Hg are usually in no immediate danger of a cardiovascular (CV) event, and drug therapy can be postponed while lifestyle modification is given a chance to work. It is well known that BP may decrease on repeated observations. This may be secondary to:

- Lifestyle interventions
- Acclimatization to the BP cuff
- A result of the "regression to the mean" phenomenon (in large groups, people at the extremes tend to gravitate to the mean or average).

There is evidence, however, to suggest that if BPs remains >140/90 mm Hg after 3 to 6 months of lifestyle intervention (as outlined in Chapter 3, *Lifestyle Modifications in the Management of Hypertension*), medication is indicated.

Some physicians and, as noted earlier, the 1999 World Health Organization—International Society of Hypertension (WHO-ISH) and the European Society of Cardiology and Society of Hypertension reports continue to advocate lifestyle management for longer periods of time without specific medication unless definite risk factors other than hypertension are present. These risk factors include:

- Diabetes
- Obesity

- Hyperlipidemia
- Evidence of coronary heart disease (CHD)
- Proteinuria.

It is well established that benefit of treatment is greatest in higher risk individuals, ie, the elderly, persons with the highest BP, or those with additional risk factors. For this reason, the Reports of the Joint National Committee (JNC) on the Prevention, Detection, Evaluation, and Treatment of High Blood Pressure and the European reports advocate more immediate therapy in these subjects but some delay in patients with lower BP and no other risk factors. For example, in a person under the age of 60 with stage 1 hypertension (140-159/90-99 mm Hg) and no other risk factors, lifestyle modifications might be continued for several months. However, if left ventricular hypertrophy (LVH) or diabetes is present, specific medical therapy in addition to lifestyle changes should be started as soon as the diagnosis is made. **Table 4.1** presents an outline of risk stratification to guide treatment decisions based on recent clinical trial evidence.

While the short or express version of JNC 7 did not specifically elaborate on risk factor classifications, it is assumed that the full report will do so, and it is also assumed that the risk factor categories will be similar to JNC-VI. However, since hypertension has now been staged as prehypertension, stage 1, and stage 2, these recommendations will most probably be somewhat modified. The European guidelines are more complicated and list risk as very high, high, moderate, and low based upon a life expectancy with various risk factors. However, the simplified guide as published by JNC-VI and modified in **Table 4.1** is still quite appropriate.

While we agree with the concept of delaying medication in low-risk individuals, physicians might be cau-

TABLE 4.1 — RISK STRATIFICATION OF HYPERTENSION TO GUIDE TREATMENT CHOICES*†

Blood Pressure Stages (mm Hg)	Initial Therapy‡		
	Risk Group A (No risk factors; no TOD/CVD)	**Risk Group B** (At least one risk factor, not including diabetes; no TOD/CVD)	**Risk Group C** (TOD or evidence of CVD and/or diabetes, with/without other risk factors)
130-139/85-89	Lifestyle modification	Lifestyle modification	Medication
140-159/90-99 (stage 1)	Lifestyle modification (3-4 months)	Lifestyle modification§ (1-3 months)	Medication
≥160/≥100 (stage 2)	Medication	Medication	Medication

Abbreviations: CVD, clinical cardiovascular disease; LVH, left ventricular hypertrophy; TOD, target-organ disease.

* Modified from JNC-VI to conform to newer definitions.

† *Lifestyle modification should be adjunctive therapy for all patients recommended for pharmacologic therapy.*

‡ For example, a patient with diabetes and a blood pressure of 142/94 mm Hg plus LVH should be classified as having stage 1 hypertension with TOD (LVH) and with another major risk factor (diabetes). Patient would be *stage 1, risk group C*; pharmacologic treatment should be initiated at the same time as lifestyle modifications.

§ For patients with multiple risk factors, clinicians should consider drugs plus lifestyle modifications as initial therapy.

55

tioned not to delay medication too long; **Table 4**.1 recognizes this concern. As noted elsewhere and in this table, we favor beginning specific medical therapy in stage 1 patients at relatively low risk somewhat earlier than some national recommendations suggest. We do not believe, for example, that patients with stage 1 hypertension should be followed for longer than 3 to 4 months even if they are <60 years of age, are nonsmokers, have a normal lipid profile, and do not have diabetes or evidence of renal or cardiac involvement.

While a majority of hypertensive patients have grade 1 or stage 1 hypertension, many of them have at least one other risk factor, including being >60 years of age. There are, therefore, a minority of hypertensive subjects who can be categorized as risk group A, with stage 1 hypertension. We should not forget the lessons from the 1930s and 1940s when all we had to offer the patient with hypertension were low-sodium diets, weight loss, phenobarbital, or mutilating surgery, such as a sympathectomy. In the days before effective therapy became available, less-severe hypertension frequently progressed to malignant or accelerated hypertension, congestive heart failure (CHF), stroke, and other complications of hypertension. These phenomena are rare today in well-treated patients. The risk for cerebrovascular and CV complications are decreased with effective BP lowering. A suggested approach to specific initial therapy is outlined in **Table 4**.2. An approach that incorporates a risk-factor assessment is outlined in **Table 4**.3.

Most patients in the low-risk group can be controlled on one medication and need not be seen by a clinician more than two or at most three times a year after BP is controlled. This approach is not costly or time consuming. To reemphasize an approach that we believe to be a reasonable one for the management of a low-risk patient with stage or grade 1 hypertension

TABLE 4.2 — SUGGESTED APPROACH TO MANAGEMENT OF A PATIENT WITH INITIAL BLOOD PRESSURE ≥140/90 MM HG*

I. BP 150-160/90-100 mm Hg

Lifestyle interventions for 3 to 4 months, depending on age and presence or absence of other risk factors:

- Weight loss if appropriate[†]
- Sodium restriction to 2 to 2.4 g/day[†]
- Exercise program (moderate and repetitive)
- Adequate intake of potassium, calcium, and magnesium
- Limit alcohol intake to less than 2 oz 80-proof whiskey, 10 oz wine, 24 oz beer (approximately one half of these amounts for women and thin individuals)
- Smoking cessation; low-fat, high-fiber diet
- Practice some form of relaxation technique.

After this period of initial observation, there are several options:[‡]

A. **BP <140/90 mm Hg:**
   Continue above—see patient in 6 months

B. **BP >140/90 mm Hg:**
   Add drug therapy

II. BP >160/100 mm Hg

Specific drug therapy plus lifestyle interventions: If after 1 year BP has remained within normal limits, medication may be reduced gradually to see if normotensive levels are maintained by nonpharmacologic means.

---

* Three readings taken a few minutes apart in the sitting position.
† Most effective nonpharmacologic interventions.
‡ See text for detailed information.

TABLE 4.3 — SUGGESTED APPROACHES FOR INITIATION OF PHARMACOLOGIC THERAPY

High Risk

- BP >140/90 mm Hg with evidence of CV disease and/or diabetes, with/without other risk factors*
- Stage 2 hypertension
- Stage 1 or 2 hypertension with at least three other risk factors*

Lifestyle modifications
and medication

Medium Risk

- Stage 1 hypertension with one other risk factor*

Lifestyle modifications for 2 to 3 months
If BP >140/90 mm Hg, begin medication

Low Risk

- Male <55 years of age
- Female <65 years of age
- Stage 1 hypertension (140-159/90-99 mm Hg) with no other risk factors*

Lifestyle modifications for 3 to 4 months
If BP >140/90 mm Hg, begin medication

Abbreviations: BP, blood pressure; CV, cardiovascular.

* Risk factors include: male >55 years of age, female >65 years of age, diabetes, smoking history, hyperlipidemia, target-organ involvement, or obesity.

and no other risk factors—lifestyle modifications for about 3 to 4 months, but if BP remains elevated, antihypertensive medication should be given and BP reduced to <140/90 mm Hg if at all possible. This may be a more aggressive treatment approach than recommended by consensus committees but is consistent with current evidence.

A Different Approach for Diabetics

As repeatedly emphasized in this book, the presence of diabetes affects the approach to treatment, even in stage 1 hypertensive patients. Diabetes should be considered a CHD equivalent rather than another CV risk factor, ie, a diabetic patient without a history or clinical findings of CHD is at a similar risk for a CV event as a nondiabetic who has evidence of CHD. Therefore, as noted, they should be treated as high-risk patients and treated pharmacologically as well as with lifestyle interventions, regardless of the level of BP elevation.

In addition, since many diabetic hypertensives also have evidence of lipid abnormalities (low high-density lipoprotein [HDL] and elevated triglyceride levels), attention should be paid to correcting these as well as reducing low-density lipoprotein (LDL) levels to <100 mg/dL with therapy similar to that suggested for patients with CHD.

Since lipid abnormalities are also common in nondiabetic hypertensives, it is important to monitor these levels; if LDL levels are >160 mg/dL, dieting and exercise interventions are suggested. If these prove ineffective in reducing LDL levels <130 mg/dL or <100 mg/dL in high-risk patients (diabetics and patients with CHD), specific medications, such as the statins or, in some cases, a statin and a fibric acid derivative, should be given. Some lipid-lowering medications will be necessary in a majority of cases. Complete guidelines for lipid management in both nondiabetic and diabetic hypertensive individuals can be found in the latest National Cholesterol Education Program report.

Beneficial Effects of Long-Term Therapy

Meta-analyses of 3- to 5-year controlled clinical trials, including trials in the elderly prior to 1997, show a high statistically significant decrease in fatal and nonfatal strokes of 38% and fatal and nonfatal coronary events of 16% compared with control or placebo groups (**Figure 4.1**). These trials achieved an average decrease of only 5-6 mm Hg diastolic blood pressure (DBP) and approximately 10-12 mm Hg systolic blood pressure (SBP) in treated groups compared with either placebo or control groups. Approximately 25% to 30% of patients did not even reach goal BP; in some instances, goal BP was set as high as DBP 95 mm Hg. Even better results might have been expected if a higher percentage of patients had been treated to a goal DBP <90 mm Hg or SBP <140 mm Hg. In the Hypertension Optimal Treatment (HOT) study in which only 8.5% of subjects ended the trial with DBP >90 mm Hg, overall CV events were lower than in previous trials (see Chapter 14, *Calcium Channel Blockers*, HOT Trial section, and **Table 14.2**.) This is in contrast to other long-term studies in which a much higher percentage of patients failed to achieve goal BP. In recent trials (Antihypertensive and Lipid-Lowering Treatment to Prevent Heart Attack Trial [ALLHAT] and Controlled Onset Verapamil Investigation of Cardiovascular End Points [CONVINCE] trial), >85% of patients achieved a goal DBP level of <90 mm Hg.

In addition to a reduction in strokes, stroke deaths, and overall CV deaths, treatment has:

- Reduced the occurrence of CHF as a complication of hypertension by more than 50%—in the 1940s, CHF accounted for about 40% of the deaths in hypertensive patients. Hypertensive heart disease is the most common cause of CHF;

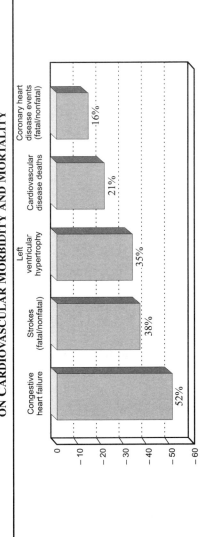

FIGURE 4.1 — EFFECT OF ANTIHYPERTENSIVE DRUG TREATMENT ON CARDIOVASCULAR MORBIDITY AND MORTALITY

Combined results from 17 randomized, placebo-controlled treatment trials; decrease in events treated compared with controls.

Arch Intern Med. 1993;153:578-581, and *J Am Coll Cardiol.* 1996;27:1214-1218.

in this era of managed care in which physicians are being urged to prevent the *recurrence* of heart failure because of the expense of repeated hospitalizations, it is important to remember that *adequate treatment of hypertension will prevent heart failure from occurring in the first place*—not in all cases, but in a sizeable number of patients.

- Prevented the occurrence of LVH or caused a regression of LVH if present prior to therapy in a large number of patients following the lowering of BP (see Chapter 17, *Results of Therapy*).
- Prevented progression from less-severe to more-severe disease, a factor not often considered. When the trials are analyzed, only 95 of 13,389 persons in treated groups compared with 1,493 of 13,342 in the placebo or control groups progressed to severe hypertension (defined as DBP ≥110-130 mm Hg and/or SBP ≥210- 230 mm Hg) (see Chapter 17, *Results of Therapy*).

There are, therefore, sufficient data to justify the treatment of hypertensive patients, even in the absence of target-organ involvement. Management should stress:

- Keeping the treatment as simple as possible
- Keeping dosages of medication low, if at all possible, to minimize side effects
- Making all efforts to increase adherence to a therapy regimen
- Treating to a goal of <140/90 mm Hg or lower in patients with diabetes or renal failure (<130/ 80-85 mm Hg); this often requires the use of two or even three medications with different modes of action.

In our experience, fewer than 10% of patients will discontinue medication because of side effects if the medications are chosen carefully and dosages kept at the lower part of the recommended range. Some studies suggest that as many as 30% to 40% of patients discontinue therapy because of side effects, but this has not been our experience, especially if low doses of different medications are used.

Factors Influencing Outcome of Therapy

Several factors determine the success of medical therapy:

- Physicians should choose a drug or drugs proven to be effective in a high percentage of patients. In our experience, the use of a diuretic will achieve goal BP in as high a percentage as other available medication when used as initial therapy, especially in black subjects or in subjects >55 years of age. One trial comparing five of the six classes of medications currently suggested as first-step or alternative therapy indicated that any of these agents lowered BP to an *almost* equivalent degree (diuretics, β-blockers, angiotensin-converting enzyme [ACE] inhibitors, calcium channel blockers [CCBs], α_1-blockers) (**Table 4.4**). In this trial, the degree of BP lowering with an ACE inhibitor (enalapril) as monotherapy was only –2.7/–1.1 mm Hg greater than with nutritional intervention. This may have occurred as a result of the population studied which included a number of black patients. It is recognized that ACE inhibitors are effective as BP-lowering agents in a wide variety of patients except for black patients, in whom they are less effective. Other comparative data from shorter-term trials suggest that the angiotensin II receptor blockers (ARBs) are as effective as the other agents.

TABLE 4.4 — AVERAGE BLOOD PRESSURE CHANGE FROM BASELINE AT 48 MONTHS IN PATIENTS IN THE TREATMENT OF MILD HYPERTENSION STUDY (TOMHS)*

	Acebutolol	Amlodipine	Chlorthalidone	Doxazosin	Enalapril	Placebo[†]
NO—	126	114	117	121	119	207
Systolic BP mm Hg change at 48 months	−13.9	−14.1	−14.6	−13.4	−11.3	−8.6
Diastolic BP mm Hg change at 48 months	−11.5	−12.2	−11.1	−11.2	−9.7	−8.6

* Baseline average blood pressure (BP) was 140/91 mm Hg. Nutritional intervention (placebo cohort) resulted in a decrease of 8.6/8.6 mm Hg in BP. Medication, in addition to lifestyle changes, resulted in an additional decrease of about 5 mm Hg systolic (except with enalapril) and about 3 mm Hg diastolic (except with enalapril). These slight additional decreases in BP resulted in an overall decrease in cardiovascular morbidity and mortality.

† Nutritional intervention only.

From: *JAMA.* 1993;270:713-724.

- BP lowering in the recently reported ALLHAT trial was greater in the diuretic-based treatment group than in an ACE inhibitor–based treatment group and essentially similar to that achieved with a CCB. Thirty-five percent of patients in this study were black.

- BP should be titrated to goal levels. Too many patients with a BP of 160/100 mm Hg, for example, are inadequately treated. BP decreases to 145-150/90-95 mm Hg and medication is not changed. If the full benefit of therapy is to be achieved, BP should be decreased to <140/90 mm Hg or as close to 120-125/80-85 mm Hg as can be achieved and tolerated by the patient. There is now good evidence that reducing BP to <130/80-85 mm Hg, if at all possible, in the diabetic patient will result in fewer CV events. In our experience, >80% of patients achieve goal BP with a simple, relatively inexpensive regimen. This frequently requires small doses of different classes of medications (eg, a diuretic plus an ACE inhibitor, an ARB, or a β-blocker). Occasionally, three different drugs may be necessary. As long as side effects are not disturbing, dosages of medications should be titrated until goal BP is achieved. As noted above, goal BP continues to be defined as <140/90 mm Hg in national and international guidelines but, based on increasing amounts of data, lower goals should be set and achieved if possible. Achieving a goal of <140 mm Hg SBP may be difficult in some elderly subjects with isolated systolic hypertension (ISH), but medication should be increased or changed until this level is reached or side effects prevent further dosage changes (see Chapter 17, *Results of Therapy*). Patients need to be seen only two or at most three times a year once BP control is achieved. This may suggest patient neglect, but good results have been achieved in the major clinical trials (eg, the Hypertension Detection and Follow-up Program [HDFP]) and in our own practice where patients were seen only three to four times a year. Follow-up visits during the first 6 months of therapy may have to be more frequent to achieve BP control.

- Patient education is important in gaining cooperation and helping patients to understand reasons for therapy. This is not the complete answer to increasing adherence to therapy, but it is helpful. We have used various patient education materials to supplement our own discussions with patients. Some booklets, *High Blood Pressure: What You Should Know About It and How You Can Help Your Doctor Treat It* and *High Blood Pressure and Diabetes—Control Them and Live Longer,* are available from Le Jacq Communications, 3 Parkland Drive, Darien, CT 06820 or can be downloaded from the Hypertension Education Foundation website (www.hypertensionfoundation.org). A great deal of "lip service" has been paid to patient education, but how often is educational material available in physicians' offices, clinics, etc? Certainly not as often as it should be.

- Occasionally, home BP recording is helpful in demonstrating to the patient that BP has been lowered. Home BP can be determined with one of the many inexpensive ($40 to $75) sphygmomanometers on the market; recent comparative studies have confirmed the accuracy of most of the electronic (digital readout) instruments. Ambulatory BP monitoring is rarely necessary.

- Keep the cost of therapy as low as possible. As many as 20% to 25% of people are unable to afford to fill their prescriptions. In addition, many become discouraged with the process of treatment when expensive diagnostic testing is used (see Chapter 2, *Diagnosis*).

The So-Called J-Shaped Curve

There is little good evidence from an analysis of the clinical trials that reducing DBP below a certain level increases CHD risk. The J-curve hypothesis suggests that since coronary arteries fill during diastole, a drop in DBP to <80-85 mm Hg in patients with coronary artery disease may decrease coronary flow and that ischemic heart disease events may actually be increased at these BP levels. This theory has been widely disseminated and has led many physicians to be concerned about decreasing BP too much, especially in the elderly. *This may account for the fact that a large number of patients with elevated SBP (ie, ISH >140 mm Hg, but with DBP <90 mm Hg) are not being treated adequately.*

These J-curve conclusions are based on small numbers of patients and extrapolation from larger sets of data, but some investigators still believe that CHD events actually increase if DBP is reduced to <80 mm Hg. But in the Systolic Hypertension in the Elderly Program (SHEP), for example, in which mean DBP was reduced to <70 mm Hg, treated patients showed a decrease, not an increase, in CHD mortality when compared with placebo subjects. Of interest in this trial, >60% of the patients had abnormal electrocardiograms (ECGs) at baseline.

On the other hand, there is some evidence from a recent reanalysis of the SHEP trial data that decreases of DBP to <55-60 mm Hg might increase CHD events, but these levels are rarely achieved in clinical practice. A prudent approach to therapy might suggest that if DBP is lowered to about 55 mm Hg, further efforts to lower SBP might be curtailed even if goal SBP has not been achieved.

The recently completed HOT study also provides no evidence that decreasing DBP to goals of 80-85 mm Hg increases risk, even in patients with ischemic heart disease. Concern about the J-curve phenomenon should not deter physicians from treating hypertension, especially in the elderly. This applies especially to individuals with ISH (elevated SBP and normal DBP).

Specific Drug Therapy

The JNC reports published periodically over the past 25 years represent the opinions of hypertension experts from across the United States. These reports are approved by medical organizations that are represented on the National High Blood Pressure Coordinating Committee of the National Heart, Lung, and Blood Institutes. After reviewing data available at the time of the JNC 7 report in 2003, the Committee concluded that "thiazide-type diuretics should be used as initial therapy for most patients with hypertension, either alone or in combination with one of the other classes (ACE inhibitors, ARBs, β-blockers, or CCBs)." This recommendation was based on evidence from long-term clinical trials that used these agents and found a significant reduction not only in cerebrovascular but in CV morbidity and mortality in treated compared with control or placebo patients. It was also based on the results of numerous comparative trials, including ALLHAT, which determined that a diuretic-based treatment program reduced morbidity and mortality to as great or greater degree than a regimen based on other medications.

Although this recommendation has been criticized by some investigators, it is quite similar to that of other JNCs which, since 1977, have consistently recommended diuretics as one of the preferred initial treatments. The objection appears to be with the designation *in most hypertensive individuals*. Part of this decision has been based upon the results of the ALLHAT study, which appeared to justify this approach. In this trial, which included >40,000 people, a diuretic-based treatment program was found to be significantly better with regard to reducing CV events (especially heart failure) when compared with an α-blocker (doxazosin). This led to the decision to recommend that an α-blocker should not be one of the preferred initial treatments.

In addition, while there was no overall difference in the primary outcome of CHD, morbidity, and mortality between the groups treated with a diuretic, an ACE inhibitor (lisinopril), or a CCB (amlodipine), there were differences in the outcome in certain subsets when the trial was completed after 5 years (>33,000 patients). For example, there were fewer incidents of significant heart failure in the diuretic-treated group compared with the amlodipine-treated group. There was also a difference in outcome with fewer strokes and overall CHF in the patients treated with the diuretic compared with lisinopril. These data led the ALLHAT investigators to conclude that diuretics were unsurpassed in their ability to reduce morbidity and mortality. The study has been criticized because of the protocol selected and the makeup of the patients studied (see Chapter 12, *ACE Inhibitors*).

Neither the ALLHAT investigators nor the JNC 7 committee concluded that ACE inhibitors, CCBs, or β-blockers were not useful, effective, and safe in the management of hypertension—only that diuretics should remain a preferred initial treatment. Another new trial, the Australian National Blood Pressure

(ANBP 2) study, which was a head-to-head comparison of a diuretic-based vs ACE inhibitor–based program, concluded that the ACE inhibitor–based program was somewhat more effective in reducing CV events than the diuretic. However, the differences were only marginally significant and only applied to males. The ANBP 2 was unblinded as compared with the ALLHAT. This study will also be critiqued in Chapter 12, *ACE Inhibitors*. The results of these two studies are not necessarily incompatible.

The JNCs 6 and 7 specifically designated special situations for the use of the following drugs (see Chapter 15, *Approach to Treatment: Combination Therapy* and **Tables 15.2** and **15.3** for details):

- ACE inhibitors
- ARBs
- CCBs
- α_1–β-Blockers
- α-Blockers
- Aldosterone antagonists.

In addition, the committees suggested that fixed-dose combinations (ie, a diuretic/β-blocker, diuretic/ACE inhibitor, diuretic/ARB, ACE inhibitor/CCB) might be appropriate initial therapy. JNC 7 reemphasized this recommendation, especially in patients with stage 2 hypertension (BP >160/100 mm Hg) or in hypertensive diabetics.

There are some specific and compelling reasons to use a given medication (**Table 4.5**). In heart failure, use an ACE inhibitor and a diuretic or an ARB or a β-blocker usually with a diuretic. An aldosterone antagonist may also be useful in these patients. If a diuretic is not being used in the treatment of ISH, it should be substituted or added to therapy. A CCB may be used if a diuretic is contraindicated or not effective. This recommendation is based on results of the Systolic

TABLE 4.5 — SOME SPECIFIC OR COMPELLING REASONS TO USE PARTICULAR MEDICATIONS*

High-Risk Conditions With Compelling Indication*	Recommended Drugs					
	Diuretic	β-Blocker	ACEI	ARB	CCB	Aldosterone Antagonist
Heart failure	✓	✓	✓	✓		✓
Post-myocardial infarction		✓	✓			✓
High coronary disease risk	✓	✓	✓	✓	✓	
Diabetes	✓	✓	✓	✓	✓	
Chronic kidney disease	✓		✓	✓		
Recurrent stroke prevention	✓		✓			

Abbreviations: ACEI, angiotensin-converting enzyme inhibitor; ARB, angiotensin II receptor blocker; CCB, calcium channel blocker.

* Compelling or specific indications for antihypertensive drugs are based on benefits from outcome studies or existing clinical guidelines.

Modified from: The JNC 7 Report. *JAMA.* 2003;289:2560-2572.

Hypertension in Europe (Syst Eur) Multicentre Trial, which reported a reduction in strokes and stroke deaths in a dihydropyridine-CCB–based trial in elderly subjects with ISH. In myocardial infarction (MI) patients, there is a strong indication to use a non-intrinsic sympathomimetic activity β-blocker; in subjects with systolic dysfunction, an ACE inhibitor or ARB is indicated.

Several outcome studies with agents other than diuretics or β-blockers have been published since 1999 and since the fifth and sixth editions of *Clinical Management of Hypertension*. Other trials have been published comparing long-term outcome results with the older drugs (diuretics and β-blockers) and the newer agents (ACE inhibitors, ARBs, and CCBs). These results are important to review again in order to clarify the reasons for recent recommendations and to emphasize that the JNC 7 recommendations are not solely based on the ALLHAT data.

There are some indications from several comparative drug trials that medications that interfere with the renin-angiotensin-aldosterone system (RAAS) (ie, ACE inhibitors and ARBs) as well as the CCBs are effective in reducing morbidity and mortality, especially if they are used with a diuretic or in combination with other agents. Long-term trials (HOT, the United Kingdom Prospective Diabetes Study [UKPDS], the Captopril Prevention Project [CAPPP]), and the Swedish Trial in Old Persons with Hypertension 2 (STOP-Hypertension-2) provide indications that treatment based on the use of long-acting CCBs or ACE inhibitors will reduce CV events (see Chapter 12, *ACE Inhibitors*, and Chapter 14, *Calcium Channel Blockers*). But the evidence suggests that results with the newer agents are not better than those with older medications (ie, diuretics/β-blockers) (see below). Overall results also suggest that a CCB-based treatment program may not be as effective as a diuretic- or diuretic/β-blocker–based regimen in reducing MI or the occurrence of heart failure. In addition, a regimen based on a RAAS blocker appears to be more effective in reducing morbidity/mortality than a CCB-based regimen, especially in diabetics or patients with renal disease.

In 2000, the Blood Pressure Lowering Treatment Trialists Collaboration performed separate meta-analyses of placebo-controlled trials in which active treatment was initiated with a calcium antagonist or an ACE inhibitor, and reported that the reduction in CV end points were similar to those found in trials in which active treatment was based on diuretics or diuretics/β-blockers. Several other analyses comprising over 67,000 randomized patients compared calcium antagonists with older drugs. For heart failure, calcium antagonists appeared to provide less protection than conventional therapy but slightly better protection against fatal and nonfatal strokes. In another analysis of five trials of >46,000 randomized patients comparing ACE inhibitors with older drugs, it was concluded that ACE inhibitors provided slightly less protection against stroke with a nonsignificant difference between the treatments for total mortality, CV mortality, all CV events, MI, etc.

Figure 4.2 and **Figure 15**.1 represent our modification of the JNC 7 recommendations. We favor the use of small doses of two different classes of drugs if monotherapy is ineffective rather than sequential monotherapy (see Chapter 15, *Approach to Treatment*: *Combination Therapy*, for details), unless BP is not lowered at all by the first agent chosen or troublesome side effects occur.

A major difference between the 1999 WHO-ISH, the European reports, and the JNC 7 report is in the recommendations for initial treatment. The WHO-ISH states that "based on recent trial evidence, there is as

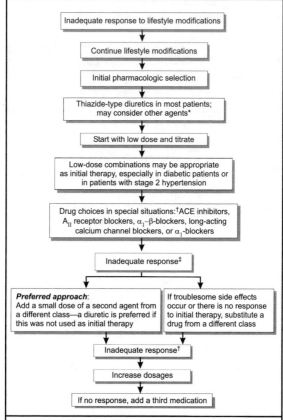

FIGURE 4.2 — MODIFICATION OF THE PHARMACOLOGIC TREATMENT ALGORITHM

Inadequate response to lifestyle modifications

Continue lifestyle modifications

Initial pharmacologic selection

Thiazide-type diuretics in most patients; may consider other agents*

Start with low dose and titrate

Low-dose combinations may be appropriate as initial therapy, especially in diabetic patients or in patients with stage 2 hypertension

Drug choices in special situations:†ACE inhibitors, A$_{II}$ receptor blockers, α_1–β-blockers, long-acting calcium channel blockers, or α_1-blockers

Inadequate response‡

Preferred approach: Add a small dose of a second agent from a different class—a diuretic is preferred if this was not used as initial therapy

If troublesome side effects occur or there is no response to initial therapy, substitute a drug from a different class

Inadequate response†

Increase dosages

If no response, add a third medication

* Calcium channel blockers may be given in some situations.
† See Figure 15.1.
‡ Response means goal blood pressure <140/90 mm Hg has been achieved or patient is making considerable progress toward this goal.

yet no evidence that the main benefits of treating hypertension are due to any particular drug property other than lowering the BP per se and that the randomized trials conducted to date have not provided any clear evidence of differential effects on outcome of different agents which produce the same BP reduction." *The committee concluded that it is probably the degree of BP lowering and not specific properties of medications that reduces morbidity and mortality in hypertensive patients.*

The European recommendations also suggested that it was reasonable to initiate therapy with any one of the five classes of medications (ie, diuretics, β-blockers, ACE inhibitors, ARBs, or CCBs). Either a low dose of a single agent or low-dose combination of two agents can be given since, especially in diabetic patients, the vast majority would require more than two drugs to produce adequate BP lowering. Additional impetus for the use of combination therapy was provided by the Perindopril Protection Against Recurrent Stroke Study (PROGRESS) in patients post–transient ischemic attack or stroke. In this trial, an ACE inhibitor as monotherapy failed to prevent recurrent stroke, but a combination of an ACE inhibitor and a diuretic was successful. The European recommendations also suggested that if low-dose monotherapy is chosen and control is not achieved, the next step is to:

- Switch to a low dose of a different agent; in other words, sequential monotherapy; or
- Increase the dose of the first compound chosen; or
- Move to combination therapy.

Thus the choices are wider than given or suggested in JNC 7. Sequential monotherapy is probably not an effective way to treat most hypertensives. The European group, unlike the WHO-ISH committee, does not recognize α-blockers as preferred initial treatment based upon the results of the ALLHAT, but nonspecifically states that α-blockers can be considered as initial therapy, particularly in combination with other drugs. The European committee recognizes that initial monotherapy is probably outdated because in most cases, two or more drugs are necessary in combination to produce goal BP.

Specific Trial Data That Have Influenced Current Treatment Recommendations

Trials that have been published that have influenced recent recommendations for therapy include:

- The STOP-Hypertension-2 and UKPDS trials appear to confirm the concept that BP lowering is more important in most instances than the drug used but, as noted, *there are exceptions.* Older agents (diuretics and/or β-blockers) produced a similar effect on morbidity and mortality as ACE inhibitors and CCBs in elderly subjects (STOP-Hypertension-2) and in the UKPDS.

- Better results regarding decreases in occurrence of MI and heart failure were noted with ACE inhibitors compared with CCBs, both in the elderly (STOP-Hypertension-2) and in diabetics (Fosinopril Versus Amlodipine Cardiovascular Events Trial [FACET] and the Appropriate Blood Pressure Control in Diabetes [ABCD] study).

- In another trial (CAPPP), the diabetic subjects in the ACE-inhibitor group had fewer CV events than those in the β-blocker group. Strokes, however, were less in the β-blocker/diuretic group. As noted, randomization was poor in this trial—higher baseline BP in the ACE-inhibitor group and more evidence of ischemic heart disease in the β-blocker group. Results must, therefore, be interpreted carefully.

- The Nordic Diltiazem (NORDIL) and the International Nifedipine Gastrointestinal Therapeutic System Study Intervention as a Goal for Hypertension Therapy (INSIGHT) studies suggest that both a nondihydropyridine CCB (diltiazem) and a dihydropyridine (nifedipine) appear to be as effective as, but no more effective than, a diuretic (NORDIL) or a β-blocker/diuretic program (INSIGHT) in reducing *overall* CV events; however, some differences were noted:
  - Fewer strokes in NORDIL with diltiazem, but a trend toward more MIs, CV deaths, and heart failure in the diltiazem group.
  - Significantly more fatal MIs and CHF with nifedipine compared with a diuretic in the INSIGHT trial (small numbers of patients).
- Three recent trials with ARBs (Reduction in End Points in Non–Insulin-Dependent Diabetes Mellitus With the Angiotensin II Antagonist Losartan [RENAAL], Irbesartan Diabetic Nephropathy Trial [IDNT], and Irbesartan Microalbuminuria II [IRMA 2]) (see Chapter 13, *Angiotensin II Receptor Blockers*) indicate that these agents are effective in reducing proteinuria and slowing progression of renal disease in type 2 diabetes.

Another trial with the ARB losartan (Losartan Intervention for End-point Reduction in Hypertension [LIFE] study) indicated that in hypertensive patients with left ventricular hypertrophy, a regimen based on the ARB was more effective in reducing overall CV events (namely, stroke) when compared with a β-blocker regimen. Physicians should consider the above results when making a choice of initial therapy.

The WHO-ISH recommendations in 1999 were consistent with data from trials at that time (**Table 4.6**), but as the report states, comparatively little information was available on the newer drugs, the α_1-blockers (prazosin, terazosin, and doxazosin), and to some extent, the ARBs (losartan, valsartan, irbesartan, telmisartan, and eprosartan). As noted, results from ALLHAT (see Chapter 10, α_1-*Adrenergic Inhibitors*) indicate that the use of α-blockers results in more CV events and especially heart failure than when diuretics are used. An α_1-blocker should not be used as initial therapy unless there is a very specific reason for its use. ALLHAT confirms previous data that the occurrence of fatal and nonfatal CHD events is similar in a diuretic-based trial as in an ACE inhibitor– or CCB-treatment regimen.

Currently it would appear, however, that ACE inhibitors and, on the basis of newer data, the ARBs have an advantage in the management of hypertensive diabetics, especially if they have renal disease. New-onset diabetes may also be reduced when these medications are used compared with other antihypertensive agents. Regimens based on the use of a RAAS inhibitor have been shown to reduce morbidity and mortality in the diabetic patient more than a CCB-based treatment program. In addition, the Heart Outcomes Prevention Evaluation (HOPE) trial indicates that an ACE inhibitor–based regimen reduced morbidity and mortality in high-risk cardiac patients more than a regimen that did not include an ACE inhibitor. A recent study, the African American Study of Kidney Disease (AASK), has also reported less progression of renal disease in patients with proteinuria when they

TABLE 4.6 — JNC 7 AND EUROPEAN RECOMMENDATIONS FOR INITIAL ANTIHYPERTENSIVE THERAPY

JNC 7	European
1. Diuretics for most patients	All available drug classes suitable for initial therapy
2. Specific indications* for: Angiotensin-converting enzyme (ACE) inhibitors β-Blockers Angiotensin II receptor blockers (ARBs) Diuretics Calcium channel blockers (CCBs)	Diuretics, β-blockers, ACE inhibitors, CCBs, and ARBs; α-blockers can be considered (usually in combination) Combination therapy may be useful in some cases
3. Low-dose combination therapy appropriate and indicated, especially in stage 2 hypertension and diabetic hypertensives	
* See Tables 15.2 and 15.3.	

From: The JNC 7 Report. *JAMA.* 2003;289:2560-2572 and 2003 European Society of Hypertension-European Society of Cardiology guidelines for the management of arterial hypertension. *J Hypertens.* 2003;21:1011-1053.

4

were treated with an ACE inhibitor or a β-blocker than with a dihydropyridine CCB.

Cost and Tolerability

Cost of therapy and adherence to or tolerability of various medications assume greater importance in making initial drug choices based on evidence of equivalence of effect in a large number of patients. These are especially important considerations for physicians as they are called upon to treat more elderly patients. While it is true, for example, that BP will be lowered effectively in hypertensive elderly individuals by long-acting CCBs, small doses of diuretics will be equally effective; cost is considerably greater with CCBs.

Well-controlled clinical trials have provided some answers to the question of tolerability to various medications. ACE inhibitors and ARBs are well tolerated by a great majority of patients but so are many of the other widely used agents when used at the lower range of recommended dosages. In the Veterans Administration double-blind comparative study and in the Treatment of Mild Hypertension Study (TOMHS), most of the drugs were well tolerated, but side effects were higher with the α-blockers when quality-of-life measurements were analyzed, regardless of the medication used first. It is often best to avoid titration beyond the initial dosage and add another agent from a different class of medication since (as noted above) the dose response curves of *most* of the antihypertensive agents are relatively flat (ie, a doubling of the dose may result in only a slight further decrease in BP but a possible increase in side effects). When ACE inhibitors or ARBs are given, there may not be an increase in adverse effects and there appears to be some additional benefit from higher doses, especially in diabetic patients or patients with heart failure.

Blood Pressure Lowering or Specific Effects of Specific Medications?

Many physicians have questioned the use of outcome studies (evidence-based medicine) as the major criterion for the selection of initial therapy, and there is some merit to this argument. Clinical judgment should also play a role, but data on morbidity and mortality outcomes are important. The WHO-ISH and European committees decided that it was the degree of BP lowering that made the difference and not specific therapy. Should we follow their advice or use clinical trial data that suggest *some* differences in outcome to guide therapy in specific cases? While most of the outcome benefits appear to derive from the degree of BP lowering (and this may also be true in the ALLHAT), I believe that the "specific benefit" data should be factored into treatment decisions. Most of the decrease in CV events in treated hypertensive patients results from the degree of BP lowering. However, there appear to be some additional benefits in certain disease states such as diabetes, renal disease, and CHD with a regimen that includes an antihypertensive medication that interferes with RAAS. The use of surrogate end points to help in our decision for initial therapy is probably of less importance.

Currently, we believe that outcome data are sufficient to guide choices, and we believe that these should continue to be a major, but not exclusive, criterion for therapy choice. Of course, in many instances the debate may be moot: *the best choice for initial therapy may be the use of small doses of two different classes of medications, one of which should be a diuretic in most cases.*

5   Diuretics

Diuretics have been used successfully since the middle 1950s in the management of hypertension. **Table 5.1** lists diuretics (available in the United States) that are used for treatment of hypertension. The duration of action varies considerably among the thiazide derivatives and other effective oral diuretic agents.

Diuretics can be divided into several classes:

- *Thiazide or thiazide-type diuretics,* which block the reabsorption of sodium in the early distal tubule
- *Indoline derivatives*
- *Loop diuretics,* which act more proximally and block sodium reabsorption in the loop of Henle (these are more potent in terms of their natriuretic effect since they act on the glomerular filtrate early in the nephron)
- *Potassium-sparing diuretics,* which act in the distal tubule, thereby preventing some of the exchange of sodium for potassium that occurs in this portion of the nephron (**Figure 5.1**).

The longer-acting thiazide diuretics are more effective as antihypertensive drugs than the loop diuretics in the dosages that are usually administered. The most commonly used diuretics in the United States are the following:

- Hydrochlorothiazide, with a duration of action of approximately 12 to 18 hours
- Chlorthalidone, with a duration of action of >24 hours
- An indoline derivative, indapamide, with a duration of action of about 18 to 24 hours.

TABLE 5.1 — DIURETICS USED FOR TREATING HYPERTENSION

Diuretic Generic (Trade) Name	Usual Dosage Range		Duration of Action (hours)	Comments
	Dose (mg)	Frequency		
Thiazides and Related Agents				
Chlorothiazide (Diuril)	125-500	1/day	24-72	More effective as antihypertensive agents than loop diuretics except in patients with serum creatinine >2.5 mg/dL—hydrochlorothiazide and chlorthalidone were used in most clinical trials
Chlorthalidone (Generic)	12.5-25	1/day	24-72	
Hydrochlorothiazide (Hydrodiuril, Microzide)	12.5-50	1/day	12-18	
Indapamide (Lozol)	1.25-2.5	1/day	18-24	A relatively low-sodium and high-potassium diet may help to augment BP lowering and prevent hypokalemia
Polythiazide (Renese)	2-4	1/day	>24	
Metolazone (Mykrox) (Zaroxolyn)	0.5-1 2.5-5	1/day 1/day	18-24	

Loop Diuretics				
Bumetanide (Bumex)	0.5-2	2/day	4-6	Not usually used as initial therapy. Higher doses may be needed for patients with renal impairment or congestive heart failure
Furosemide (Lasix)	20-80	2/day	6-8	
Torsemide (Demadex)	2.5-10	1/day*	6-12+	Long duration of action may make this more suitable for treatment of hypertensive patients
Potassium-Sparing Diuretics				
Amiloride (Midamor)	5-10	1 or 2/day	18-24	Weak diuretics when given alone—used mainly in combination with other diuretics to avoid or reverse hypokalemia; avoid when serum creatinine >2.5 mg/dL or in patients receiving an angiotensin-converting enzyme (ACE) inhibitor or an angiotensin II receptor blocker (ARB); may cause hyperkalemia
Triamterene (Dyrenium)	50-100	1 or 2/day	7-9	
Aldosterone Antagonists				
Eplerenone (Inspra)	50-100	1 or 2/day	4-6	Similar precautions as for potassium-sparing agents; more effective in lowering BP
Spironolactone (Aldactone)	25-50	2 or 3/day	8-12	
* Effect on blood pressure (BP) is longer than with other loop diuretics.				

5

FIGURE 5.1 — SITE OF ACTION OF DIURETICS

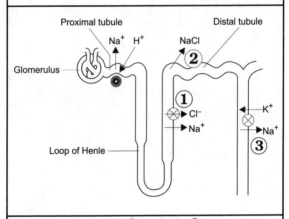

Key: ① loop diuretics, ② thiazides, ③ potassium-sparing agents.

Potassium-sparing diuretics are usually not used by themselves; they are weak diuretics and are relatively ineffective in lowering blood pressure (BP) when used alone. Various combinations of thiazides and potassium-sparing agents are available (eg, Dyazide, Maxzide, Moduretic).

The aldosterone antagonists, spironolactone and eplerenone, are more effective as BP-lowering agents than the potassium-sparing diuretics.

Mechanism of Action

The exact mechanism of action of diuretics in lowering BP is not known, although they have been used for 40-plus years. Initially, there is a decrease in plasma volume with a lowering of BP and a short-term decrease in cardiac output. Over time, however:

- Cardiac output returns to normal levels
- BP remains low

- Plasma volume returns to just slightly below pretreatment levels
- Vascular resistance decreases.

The ultimate effect of thiazide or thiazidelike diuretic therapy is reduction of arterial resistance both at rest and after exercise. The long-term effect is one of vasodilation; some recent data suggest that vasodilation is actually a primary effect of diuretics and may be related to their effect on potassium channels. With a persistent reduction of plasma volume, however, the renin-angiotensin-aldosterone system (RAAS) continues to be stimulated (**Figure 5.2**). This effect is not usually great enough to negate diuretic-induced vasodilation and BP reduction. In nonresponders, however, counteracting the activation of the RAAS by the addition of a β-blocker, angiotensin-converting enzyme (ACE) inhibitor, or angiotensin II receptor blocker (ARB) will increase BP-lowering effects. **Figure 5.3** summarizes these actions.

Approximately 50% to 60% of patients will respond to diuretics as monotherapy even when they are given in relatively small doses. As with many antihypertensive agents, the dose-response curve of diuretics is relatively flat. In people who respond to a diuretic, a dose of 12.5 mg hydrochlorothiazide or its equivalent will reduce BP in approximately one half to two thirds of them. Increasing the dose to 25 mg will add another 10% to 15% to the responders. At 50 mg hydrochlorothiazide or its equivalent, probably 80% to 90% of possible responders will experience a BP decrease. A dose of 100 mg may add a few patients to the response list or decrease the BP to a slightly greater extent, but probably at the cost of additional side effects. This is why we believe that it is more appropriate to give a small or moderate dose of a diuretic; if this does not achieve normotensive lev-

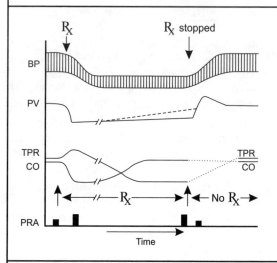

FIGURE 5.2 — HEMODYNAMIC EFFECTS OF CHLOROTHIAZIDE IN A HYPERTENSIVE PATIENT

Abbreviations: BP, blood pressure; CO, cardiac output; PV, plasma volume; PRA, plasma-renin activity; R_x, drug therapy; TPR, total peripheral resistance.

After about 4 to 6 weeks of treatment, BP remains below pretreatment levels, CO has returned to normal, and vascular resistance is reduced, but PV remains slightly below pretreatment levels. TPR and BP return to pretreatment levels when the diuretic is stopped.

From: *Circulation.* 1970;41:709-717.

els of BP, a small dose of another drug from another class (eg, ACE inhibitor, ARB, or β-blocker) should be added rather than increasing the diuretic dose still further. As noted, these other medications will block or interfere with some of the homeostatic mechanisms activated by the diuretic's effect on the RAAS. We prefer this approach to therapy with the use of small doses

FIGURE 5.3 — PHYSIOLOGIC EFFECTS OF DIURETICS

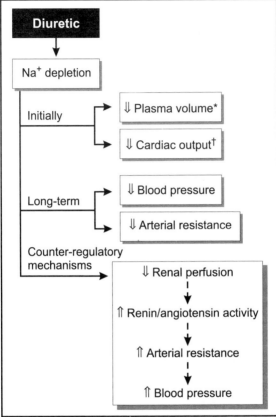

The ultimate result of diuretic therapy is reduction of arterial resistance and blood pressure. However, a continuing increase in the activity of the renin-angiotensin system is noted. *This does not, in most cases, negate the blood pressure response,* but can be counteracted in nonresponsive patients by the addition of small doses of an angiotensin-converting enzyme (ACE) inhibitor, a β-blocker, or an angiotensin II receptor blocker.

* Returns to near normal levels after several weeks.
† Returns to normal after several weeks.

of different agents, regardless of which medication is used initially, rather than titrating one drug to a high dose and then trying another (sequential monotherapy). A more complete review of therapy will be outlined in Chapter 15, *Approach to Treatment: Combination Therapy*.

Studies have shown that diuretics decrease BP by approximately 10-15/5-10 mm Hg more than placebo. The effect is consistently greater on systolic blood pressure than on diastolic blood pressure, an important point to remember in the treatment of elderly subjects in whom isolated systolic hypertension may be present.

Side Effects

Diuretics are as well tolerated as any of the other antihypertensive drugs. In the double-blind comparative Veterans Administration Study and the Treatment of Mild Hypertension Study (TOMHS), only about 3% of patients on these agents withdrew because of side effects. This was the lowest percentage of any of the other five classes of drugs tested against placebo. The most annoying side effect of diuretic therapy is sexual dysfunction, which, in our experience, occurs in about 5% to 10% of patients. This occurs most frequently in men, but can also be seen in women in the form of decreased libido and delay in orgasm. It can sometimes be attenuated by:

- Decreasing the dosage
- Using therapy on alternate days
- Omitting the drug for 2 or 3 days at a time.

Sexual dysfunction may cease to be a problem when the diuretic is stopped. But since this problem often occurs in men who are ≥60 years of age, there may not be an improvement in impotence or loss of libido when the diuretic is discontinued (ie, medication may have had nothing to do with the dysfunction). Data from TOMHS suggest that a high percentage of hypertensive patients have some sexual dysfunction prior to specific therapy. The availability of effective oral medication to improve erectile dysfunction has helped alleviate this problem in men.

In men with symptomatic prostatic hypertrophy, symptoms may be worsened. Urinary frequency or urgency may be of sufficient severity to warrant the use of another medication, but the use of small doses of a diuretic will usually not result in a significant problem. If symptoms of prostatism are severe, the use of an α-blocker (doxazosin or terazosin) will usually be helpful. Skin rash or photosensitivity is rare; pancreatitis is extremely rare but can occur.

The significance of the metabolic changes that may occur with the use of diuretics has been debated for many years (**Table 5.2**). In our opinion, the negative aspects of these have been overstated. It is important to clarify this issue.

■ Hypokalemia

Approximately 30% of patients will experience a decrease in serum potassium of about 0.5 to 0.8 mEq/L on doses of 50 to 100 mg/day hydrochlorothiazide or its equivalent. This change is dose related; on lower doses of 25 mg, the decrease is usually <0.3 to 0.4 mEq/L. In the Antihypertensive and Lipid-Lowering Treatment to Prevent Heart Attack Trial (ALLHAT), which used 12.5 to 25.0 mg/day of chlorthalidone, there was a decrease in potassium from 4.3 mEq/L to 4.1 mEq/L at 4 years. In the calcium channel blocker (CCB) and ACE inhibitor groups, potassium levels rose from 4.3 to 4.4 mEq/L to 4.4 to 4.5 mEq/L, respectively. Eight percent of patients experienced a decrease in serum potassium levels to <3.5 mEq/L on the diuretic compared with 2% and 1% on the CCB or ACE inhibitor, respectively. Reports that

TABLE 5.2 — POTENTIAL METABOLIC CHANGES WITH DIURETIC USE	
Metabolic Change	**Comments**
Hypokalemia	Less marked with lower dosages; avoid if possible, especially in diabetics and patients receiving digitalis
Hyperlipidemia	*Short term*—an increase of 5% to 7% in total cholesterol and low-density lipoproteins (may be less with smaller doses); no effect on high-density lipoproteins. *Long term—little effect*—cardiovascular events reduced to the same degree in subjects with hyperlipidemia or normal cholesterol levels
Increased insulin resistance	Insulin resistance increased. But only slight increase in blood glucose levels in long-term trials in diuretic-treated compared with placebo subjects. A 0.6% to 3.5% increase in new-onset diabetes when compared with other medications. Overall cardiovascular mortality reduced to same or greater degree in diabetics than in nondiabetics
Hyperuricemia	Gout in about 3% of patients; if diuretic essential to management, allopurinol can be given
Hypercalcemia	May be advantage in treatment of osteoporosis and prevention of fractures

diuretic-induced hypokalemia resulted in increased ectopy, ventricular tachycardia, or sudden death have not been confirmed by prospective repeated 24- and 48-hour Holter monitor studies. These have shown that, despite the occurrence of hypokalemia, there was little increase in single ventricular premature beats, couplets, or episodes of ventricular tachycardia (**Table 5.3**). Hypokalemia should be avoided, however, if possible, especially in:

- Elderly patients
- Patients on digitalis
- Patients with diabetes where the degree of hypokalemia may affect insulin utilization.

5

We therefore tend to use a potassium-sparing thiazide combination as initial therapy in such patients. This does not add significantly to cost and eliminates the need for potassium supplements or careful monitoring. Normokalemia is not, however, achieved in all cases, especially if high doses of the diuretic are used.

Many of the available thiazide and potassium-sparing combination agents actually contain a small amount of the thiazide component (12.5 mg to a maximum of 50 mg or the equivalent of hydrochlorothiazide [HCTZ]). BP lowering is maintained, and metabolic changes are minimized. *In the dosages now recommended for most of the orally effective diuretics, low potassium levels are not usually a problem.* In fixed-dose combinations with β-blockers, ACE inhibitors and ARBs, doses of 6.25 mg or 12.5 mg HCTZ greatly increase the BP-lowering effects of the other agents with a minimal effect on potassium.

The use of eplerenone, an aldosterone antagonist that has fewer side effects than spironolactone, will lower BP without causing a decrease in potassium levels. The aldosterone antagonists act to inhibit the aldosterone-mediated exchange of sodium and potas-

TABLE 5.3 — VENTRICULAR ECTOPY IN PATIENTS WITH OR WITHOUT LEFT VENTRICULAR HYPERTROPHY BEFORE AND AFTER HYDROCHLOROTHIAZIDE* (50 TO 100 MG/DAY FOR 4 WEEKS)

	LVH (n = 28)		No LVH (n = 16)	
	Baseline	Diuretic	Baseline	Diuretic
LVPWT	1.39	—	1.03	—
PK (mEq/L)	4.06	3.39	4.10	3.33
PVC/h	16.6	10.1	2.1	3.0
Total couplets	123.0	15.0	6.0	3.0
Total VT episodes	5.0	3.0	2.0	0.0

Abbreviations: LVH, left ventricular hypertrophy; LVPWT, left ventricular posterior wall thickness; PK, plasma potassium; PVC, premature ventricular contractions; VT, ventricular tachycardia.

* No increase in ectopy following high-dose diuretic therapy in subjects with or without LVH.

From: *Arch Intern Med.* 1988;148:1272.

sium in the distal tubules. This prevents potassium wastage, which may occur with a thiazide diuretic. Although data on combination therapy with a thiazide diuretic are limited, this combination, which is not currently available, will probably prove to be highly effective. In addition to BP-lowering effects, the aldosterone antagonists may inhibit myocardial fibrosis, angiogenesis induced by fibroblast growth factor, and endothelial thickening after vascular injury.

It is of interest to note that in the Systolic Hypertension in the Elderly Program (SHEP), coronary events were not reduced to the same degree in patients who experienced a serum potassium of <3.5 mEq/L as they were in other patients. Although outcome was not worsened compared with placebo, these data indicate that outcome benefit with regard to CV events was greater in patients who maintained a relatively normal potassium level on thiazide diuretics. Similar findings were noted in the Heart Outcomes Prevention Evaluation (HOPE) trial, in which outcome in patients with hypokalemia was significantly worse ($P = 0.02$) compared with patients who remained normokalemic.

■ **Effects on Lipids**

Thiazide diuretics may increase serum cholesterol levels by about 5% to 7% within the first 3 to 12 months of therapy. The effect on high-density lipoprotein (HDL) cholesterol is minimal or nonexistent; low-density lipoprotein (LDL) cholesterol increases parallel the effect on total cholesterol. However, in the 3- to 5-year clinical trials, there is little or no change in cholesterol levels following the use of even high-dose diuretic therapy (**Table 5.4**). In most of the studies, there was actually a decrease in cholesterol levels over time, especially in those patients with hyperlipidemia; this latter change may be secondary to "regression to the mean."

TABLE 5.4 — EFFECT OF DIURETIC-BASED THERAPY ON SERUM CHOLESTEROL IN LONG-TERM CLINICAL TRIALS*

Trial	Duration	Total cholesterol level (mg/dL)			Difference
		Baseline	Medication		
Berglund & Anderson	6 yrs	267	255		–12
MRC Trial: Men/Women — active treatment	3+ yrs	245/261	245/260		0/–1
— placebo		244/260	239/256		–5/–4
MAPHY	6 yrs	244	243		–1
HDFP (stepped-care [SC] group); relatively high doses of diuretics	4 yrs	232	223		–9
Oslo — active treatment/control	4 yrs	272/278	273/280		+1/+2
MRFIT — special intervention (SI) group	6 yrs	254	236		–18
— unusual care (UC) group		254	240		–14
HAPPHY Trial	4 yrs	242	242		—
EWPHE — active treatment/placbo	3 yrs	256/259	238/239		–18/–20

MRC in Elderly — active treatment/placebo	5 yrs	228/228	232/232	+4/+4
Jeunemâtre, et al	20 mos	228	232	+4
TOMHS — active treatment/placebo	2 yrs	231/235	226.5/219.9	−4.5/−5.1
VA Multi-drug	2 yrs	†	—	—
SHEP	3 yrs	2.1‡	5.3‡	3.2§
ALLHAT — diuretic	5+ yrs	216	197	−19‖

Abbreviations: ACE, angiotensin-converting enzyme; ALLHAT, Antihypertensive and Lipid-Lowering Treatment to Prevent Heart Attack Trial; CCB, calcium channel blocker; EWPHE, European Working Party on High Blood Pressure in the Elderly; HAPPHY, Heart Attack Primary Prevention in Hypertension; HDFP, Hypertension Detection and Follow-up Program; MAPHY, Metoprolol Atherosclerosis Prevention in Hypertension Study; MRC, Medical Research Council; MRFIT, Multiple Risk Factor Intervention Trial; SHEP, Systolic Hypertension in the Elderly Program; TOMHS, Treatment of Mild Hypertension Study; VA, Veterans Administration.

* Most of the trials used diuretics in doses equivalent to ≥50 mg/day of hydrochlorothiazide.
† No significant difference between diuretics and other drug treatment vs placebo.
‡ Changes from baseline.
§ Difference between placebo and active-treatment group.
‖ Decrease of −21 with ACE inhibitor; decrease of −21 with CCB (many of these patients in all three groups were also receiving statins).

Modified and updated from: *Cleve Clin J Med.* 1993;60:27-37.

For example, in the Hypertension Detection and Follow-up Program (HDFP), which used diuretics as baseline therapy, cholesterol levels in patients who entered the study with levels of ≥280 mg/dL decreased, those in patients at levels of 200 mg/dL increased slightly, and those in patients in the 220 to 230 mg/dL range remained essentially the same over a 5-year period (**Figure 5.4**). In the 2-year Verapamil in Hypertension Atherosclerosis Study (VHAS), which compared sustained-release verapamil (CCB) to chlorthalidone, serum cholesterol levels were reduced from 224 to 217 mg/dL in the chlorthalidone group. Changes did not differ from those noted with the lipid-neutral

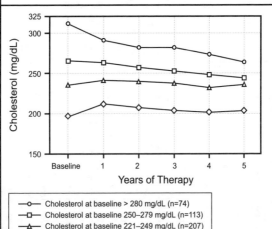

FIGURE 5.4 — EFFECT OF DIURETIC-BASED THERAPY ON CHOLESTEROL LEVELS IN THE HYPERTENSION DETECTION AND FOLLOW-UP PROGRAM (HDFP) STUDY

Subjects with pretreatment levels >280 mg/dL experienced a decrease (see text).

From: *JAMA*. 1979;242:2562.

CCB. Thus there is little evidence that diuretics should be avoided in patients with hyperlipidemia if these medications are necessary to lower BP. As noted, there is also little evidence to suggest that any short-term effect on lipids counteracts the beneficial effects of the lowering of BP; coronary heart disease events have been decreased to a statistically significant degree in diuretic-based therapy programs.

In the SHEP and HDFP studies, both of which were diuretic based, morbidity and mortality for cardiovascular (CV) diseases were reduced to the same degree in patients with baseline low and high serum cholesterol levels.

At 4 years in ALLHAT which compared a thiazide-based treatment program (chlorthalidone) with one based on an ACE inhibitor (lisinopril) or a CCB (amlodipine), the difference between groups was about 2 mg/dL (a decrease from 216 to 197 mg/dL in the chlorthalidone group; a decrease from 217 to 196 and from 216 to 195 in the CCB and ACE inhibitor groups, respectively). The results of this trial, however, were affected by the fact that a large percentage of patients were receiving statins.

■ **Insulin Resistance**

Some but not all published data indicate that insulin resistance is increased in diuretic-treated patients, whereas with some other therapies, such as ACE inhibitors, insulin resistance may not change or may actually improve. The clinical significance of this finding awaits further clarification. Serum glucose levels in the 3- to 5-year clinical trials were increased to only a slight degree (**Table 5.5**), and there was only a minimal increase in the incidence of new-onset diabetes (admittedly, none of the trials were designed to look specifically at this issue). As noted, these trials were diuretic based but also used other agents such as β-blockers or centrally acting agents to lower BP.

TABLE 5.5 — EFFECTS OF MODERATE- AND HIGH-DOSE DIURETIC THERAPY ON GLUCOSE METABOLISM

Study	Duration/Years	Serum Glucose (mg/dL)	Hyperglycemia or Diabetes
Oslo	5	No difference——diuretics; placebo	No specific data available
EWPHE	3	Increase 6.6—diuretics; placebo	Excess of 6/1000 patient years
MRC	3	No specific data available	Excess of 6/1000 patient years
HAPPHY	4	No specific data available	Excess of 6/1000 patient years
HDFP	5	No specific data available	1.6% (57/3563)
SHEP	3	Difference of 4 mg/dL—drug vs placebo in diabetics	1 of 483
	3	Difference of 3 mg/dL in nondiabetics	No significant difference in number of new cases of diabetes in treatment group compared with placebo group
MRFIT	6	No specific data available	Excess of 7%—special intervention group with diuretics vs excess of 2%—usual care group without diuretics*

ALLHAT	at 4+ years		Increase of 3 mg/dL (ACE inhibitor ↓ 1 mg/dL)	3.5% more new-onset diabetes with diuretics compared with ACE inhibitors[†]
VA	2		Increase of 1.7—diuretics; placebo	No specific data available
TOMHS	1		Decrease of 0.9—diuretics Decrease of 3.2—placebo	No specific data available

Abbreviations: ACE, angiotensin-converting enzyme; ALLHAT, Antihypertensive and Lipid-Lowering Treatment to Prevent Heart Attack Trial; EWPHE, European Working Party on High Blood Pressure in the Elderly; HAPPHY, Heart Attack Primary Prevention in Hypertension; HDFP, Hypertension Detection and Follow-up Program; MRC, Medical Research Council; MRFIT, Multiple Risk Factor Intervention Trial; SHEP, Systolic Hypertension in the Elderly Program; TOMHS, Treatment of Mild Hypertension Study; VA, Veterans Administration single-drug therapy for hypertension in men.

* Fasting glucose ≥110 mg/dL.
† Fasting glucose >126 mg/dL.

Modified and updated from: *Cleve Clin J Med.* 1993;60:27-37.

5

101

In ALLHAT, the definition of new-onset diabetes was different from that in previous trials >126 mg/dL compared with >140 mg/dL, respectively. The exception was the MRFIT trial in which a fasting glucose level of >110 mg/dL was considered to be elevated (**Table 5.5**). In ALLHAT, there was a 3.5% increase in new-onset diabetes in patients on diuretics compared with a group of patients treated with an ACE inhibitor (an increase of 3 mg/dL was noted at 4 years compared with a decrease of 1 mg/dL in serum glucose levels in the diuretic and ACE-inhibitor groups, respectively).

One could argue that since insulin resistance is increased in many hypertensive patients before therapy, any medication that might make this worse should be avoided. It might have been expected, therefore, that in the outcome trials in middle-aged or older patients with pretreatment abnormalities in insulin resistance who were exposed to a medication that had a significant effect on glucose metabolism, new-onset diabetes would have occurred more frequently, even in the relatively short 3- to 5-plus–year time period of these studies.

Recent data have demonstrated that:

- Diabetics treated with diuretics experience as great or greater decrease in coronary heart disease events and mortality than nondiabetics (**Figure 5.5**). In the United Kingdom Prospective Diabetes Study (UKPDS), in which more than 1000 hypertensive type 2 diabetic subjects were followed for more than 8 years, CV events were reduced equally in an ACE inhibitor–based program compared with one that was β-blocker/diuretic–based *if* BP was reduced, ie, the BP difference, not the specific therapy used, accounted for the benefit.

- In a follow-up of a large number of hypertensive patients, those treated with diuretics did not

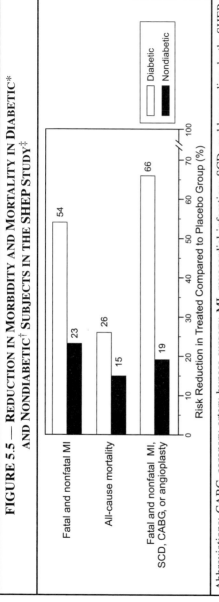

FIGURE 5.5 — REDUCTION IN MORBIDITY AND MORTALITY IN DIABETIC* AND NONDIABETIC[†] SUBJECTS IN THE SHEP STUDY[‡]

Risk Reduction in Treated Compared to Placebo Group (%)

□ Diabetic
■ Nondiabetic

Fatal and nonfatal MI — 54 / 23

All-cause mortality — 26 / 15

Fatal and nonfatal MI, SCD, CABG, or angioplasty — 66 / 19

Abbreviations: CABG, coronary artery bypass surgery; MI, myocardial infarction; SCD, sudden cardiac death; SHEP, Systolic Hypertension in the Elderly Program Cooperative Research Group.

* Therapy group = 283 subjects, placebo group = 300 subjects.
† Therapy group = 2,080 subjects, placebo group = 2,069 subjects.
‡ Low-dose diuretic as initial therapy; β-blocker added if necessary.

go on to require antidiabetic therapy any more frequently than did patients treated with ACE inhibitors, β-adrenergic inhibitors, CCBs, or α_1-blockers (**Figure 5.6**). Thus in this study, there was little evidence that diuretics should not be used if these agents are necessary to lower BP.

Several other recent studies, including ALLHAT, have noted that new-onset diabetes is less frequent in patients treated with a regimen that includes an agent that interferes with the RAAS.

The Captopril Prevention Project (CAPPP) that compared an ACE inhibitor–based regimen to that of a β-blocker/diuretic–based program reported that the

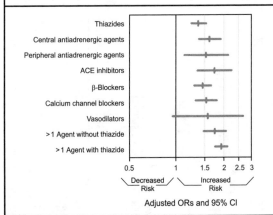

FIGURE 5.6 — RISK OF HYPERGLYCEMIA WITH USE OF ANTIHYPERTENSIVE DRUGS

Risk for development of hyperglycemia requiring treatment with antidiabetic drugs in users of antihypertensive drugs relative to nonusers. Note increased risk overall in hypertensive subjects compared with nonhypertensives, but no difference between drugs.

From: *Ann Intern Med.* 1993;118:273-278.

incidence of new-onset diabetes was less in the ACE inhibitor group. A considerable number of subjects in the ACE inhibitor cohort required a diuretic to lower BP to goal levels. As noted, there were problems with randomization in this trial.

Based on data from these trials, the preferred treatment in obese hypertensive subjects or in those with a family history of diabetes might be a small dose of a diuretic with an ACE inhibitor as initial therapy.

Both serum lipids and blood glucose levels should be checked approximately 3 to 6 months after initiating therapy with a diuretic to detect those few patients who may experience some significant changes in these metabolic parameters. If such a change is noted, a more careful follow-up may be necessary. This extra blood test will not add significantly to treatment cost and represents good medical care in the treatment of a hypertensive individual, regardless of the medication used.

■ Hyperuricemia

Large doses of thiazide diuretics (50 to 100 mg/day) increase serum uric acid levels by about 0.8 to 1.5 mg/dL and, in about 3% of patients, precipitate gouty attacks. The effect on uric acid is attenuated with the smaller doses that are now used compared with those previously recommended in the 1980s. With doses currently suggested as initial therapy by the Joint National Committees (JNCs) (approximately 12.5 mg or 25 mg of hydrochlorothiazide, 12.5 mg of chlorthalidone, 1.25 mg to 2.5 mg of indapamide), the incidence of gout is lower than it was in the early clinical trials in which doses of 50 to 100 mg/day were routinely given. If it is important to regulate BP with a diuretic and uric acid levels rise to >10 mg/dL or gout occurs, the use of allopurinol in doses of 100 to 300 mg/day has generally been effective in reducing the level of hyperuricemia and preventing gout. Whether a diuretic-induced elevation in uric acid levels poses an increased risk of a CV event has not been established.

■ Hypercalcemia

Hypercalcemia may also occur in a small number of patients because the use of diuretics results in calcium retention. This has not proved to be a problem; however, in some instances, it has led to additional testing to rule out hyperparathyroidism. An elevation of calcium levels may represent an advantage in some osteoporotic individuals, especially postmenopausal women. There is some evidence that the use of thiazide diuretics will prevent osteoporosis and fractures.

Combination Diuretics With Other Medications

We have always believed that diuretics should be one of the preferred initial monotherapies and the JNC 7 committee has recommended that a thiazidelike diuretic should represent initial therapy in most hypertensives unless there is a specific or compelling reason to use another medication. If a diuretic is not chosen as initial therapy or proves only partially effective, it should be combined with one of the other antihypertensive medications. When used in combination with a small dose of a β-adrenergic inhibitor, an ACE inhibitor, an ARB, or a CCB, response to normotensive levels is approximately 75% to 80%.

Many effective combination thiazide or other diuretic preparations are available (**Table 5.6**). Recent data indicate that combination therapies that contain a diuretic may be more effective than those that do not.

Indoline Derivatives

Indapamide (Lozol) is an effective, long-acting diuretic with a chemical composition that differs from that of the thiazides. It is well tolerated and acceptable as a substitute for any of the thiazide diuretics. In the low doses of 1.25 to 2.5 mg/day currently recommended, any metabolic changes (even short-term) are minimal. Recent trials with indapamide have demonstrated that in patients with transient ischemic attacks (TIAs) or a history of stroke without severe disability, the BP reduction of only 5/2 mm Hg reduced the incidence of total stroke over a 3-year period. Results were similar in normotensive and hypertensive patients. A combination of an ACE inhibitor and indapamide (perindopril plus indapamide) is available and is an effective antihypertensive agent.

The Perindopril Protection Against Recurrent Stroke Study (PROGRESS) reported that BP lowering with a regimen of this ACE inhibitor plus indapamide reduced the recurrence of stroke by 28% and the incidence of all CV events by 26% in normotensive and hypertensive patients with a history of stroke or TIA. Of interest in this study is that results for the ACE inhibitor alone were not statistically significantly different than those for placebo. However, the combination of the ACE inhibitor and the diuretic resulted in dramatic decreases in recurrent stroke.

Loop Diuretics

Loop diuretics (ie, furosemide, bumetanide, and torsemide) are usually reserved for patients:

- Whose creatinine levels are >2 mg % (ie, cases in which thiazide diuretics may not be effective)
- With congestive heart failure.

TABLE 5.6 — Thiazide Combination Therapies (Other Than Potassium-Sparing Diuretics)

Generic Name	Trade Name	Lowest Dose Available (mg) (Drug/Thiazide)
Atenolol + chlorthalidone	Tenoretic	50/25
Benazepril + thiazide	Lotensin HCT	5/6.25
Bisoprolol + thiazide*	Ziac	2.5/6.25
Candesartan + thiazide	Atacand HCT	16/12.5
Captopril + thiazide*	Capozide	25/15
Clonidine + chlorthalidone	Clorpres	0.1/15
Enalapril + thiazide	Vaseretic	5/12.5
Eprosartan + thiazide	Teveten HCT	600/12.5
Fosinopril + thiazide	Monopril HCT	10/12.5
Irbesartan + thiazide	Avalide	150/12.5
Lisinopril + thiazide	Prinzide, Zestoretic	10/12.5
Losartan + thiazide	Hyzaar	50/12.5

Metoprolol + thiazide	Lopressor HCT	50/25
Methyldopa + thiazide	Aldoril	250/15
Moexipril + thiazide	Uniretic	7.5/12.5
Nadolol + bendroflumethiazide	Corzide	40/5
Olmesartan + thiazide	Benicar HCT	20/12.5
Quinapril + thiazide	Accuretic	10/12.5
Propranolol + thiazide	Inderide	80/50
Prazosin + polythiazide	Minizide	1/0.5
Reserpine + chlorthalidone	Diupres	0.125/25
Reserpine + thiazide	Hydropres	0.125/25
Telmisartan + thiazide	Micardis HCT	40/12.5
Timolol + thiazide	Timolide	10/25
Valsartan + thiazide	Diovan HCT	80/12.5

* Approved as initial once-a-day therapy.

These are highly effective diuretics, but in commonly used doses given 2 to 3 times daily, they may not lower BP as much as the longer-acting diuretics. The short duration of action of most of the loop diuretics may explain this effect. *Torsemide* (Demadex) is a longer-acting loop diuretic; BP control has been demonstrated 18 to 24 hours after a single dose. This medication may be as effective on a once-a-day basis in lowering BP as a thiazide.

Metolazone (Zaroxolyn) is a longer-acting, potent diuretic that acts near the proximal tubule; it is effective in the presence of renal insufficiency. We often combine its use in small doses of 1 to 2 mg/day with furosemide or one of the other loop diuretics in difficult-to-manage hypertensive patients with renal disease.

6 β-Adrenergic Receptor Blockers

β-Adrenergic receptor blockers inhibit the effect of β-adrenergic stimuli on various organs. *Stimulation* of β-adrenergic receptors results in:

- Renin release
- Vasodilation
- Bronchodilation
- An increase in pulse rate and cardiac output
- Various metabolic effects, such as:
  - An increase in insulin secretion
  - Glycogenolysis
  - Gluconeogenesis in both the liver and the skeletal muscle.

β-Blockers block these effects to various degrees, depending on the specific drug used and the type of β-adrenergic receptor that is inhibited. For example, they tend to induce:

- Vasoconstriction
- Bronchoconstriction
- *A decrease in:*
  - Pulse rate
  - Cardiac output
  - Myocardial oxygen demand
  - Blood pressure (BP)
  - Renin release, angiotensin II, and aldosterone production.

This latter action is often forgotten; β-blockers effectively reduce the activity of the renin-angiotensin-aldosterone system (RAAS).

Obviously, the tendency to produce vasoconstriction is not desirable in hypertension, but the net effects of the other actions of β-blockers result in a decrease in BP.

There are several types of β-blockers available (**Table 6.1**). Acebutolol, atenolol, betaxolol, bisoprolol, and metoprolol are more active in inhibiting the action of β_1-receptors on cardiac muscle (cardiac selectivity) as well as other smooth muscle sites than β_2-receptors, which affect mainly peripheral vessels and bronchial smooth muscle. Of these agents, bisoprolol appears to possess the greatest degree of cardioselectivity, which theoretically limits β_2-blocker effects on pulmonary function and peripheral vessels. Most investigators, however, agree that even these agents should not be used or should only be used with care in:

- Patients with asthma where even a partial blockade of β_2-agonists may increase asthma
- Patients with severe peripheral arterial disease where any degree of blockade of β_2-receptors will leave α- or vasoconstrictor receptors unopposed, making peripheral arterial disease worse
- Patients with Raynaud's phenomenon
- Possibly patients with insulin-dependent diabetes, where symptoms of an insulin reaction such as tachycardia may be blocked, an occurrence that is less common than formerly believed.

In general, the cardioselective agents will cause less of a decrease in peripheral arterial flow or pulmonary air movement than nonselective agents, but none are completely "cardioselective."

β-Blockers presumably lower BP by:
- Decreasing cardiac output
- Inhibiting the release of renin and the production of angiotensin II

- Possibly reducing norepinephrine release from sympathetic neurons
- Decreasing central vasomotor activity.

Some β-adrenergic inhibitors, such as pindolol or acebutolol, that have some β_2-agonist or stimulating properties (intrinsic sympathomimetic activity [ISA]) may lower BP without:
- Reducing cardiac output
- Producing significant bradycardia.

They may also have less of an effect on peripheral resistance; cold extremities are reportedly less common as a side effect. In our experience, however, these agents may be less effective as BP-lowering drugs, at least in the doses that we have used (pindolol up to 15 to 20 mg/day, acebutolol up to 400 to 600 mg/day). They are indicated, however, in treating patients with angina or hypertension who have a resting bradycardia, where an additional decrease in heart rate might produce deleterious effects. There are no long-term studies of these specific agents to determine their protective effects in patients with coronary heart disease (CHD).

There are also differences in β-blockers regarding their lipid solubility. Those agents that are lipid soluble:
- Cross the blood-brain barrier
- Are reported to produce more central nervous system (CNS) effects
- Have a shorter duration of action since they are inactivated more rapidly by the liver ("first-pass" phenomenon).

Propranolol (Inderal LA and InnoPran XL) and metoprolol (Lopressor) are examples of lipid soluble antihypertensive β-blockers.

Atenolol (Tenormin) and nadolol (Corgard) are examples of agents that are less lipid-soluble; for example:
- Smaller amounts reach the CNS

TABLE 6.1 — β-BLOCKERS USED FOR TREATING HYPERTENSION*

Generic (Trade) Name	Usual Dosage Range*		Physiologic Effects	Comments
	Dose (mg)	Frequency		
Atenolol† (Tenormin)	25-100	1/day	→ cardiac output; → plasma renin activity; → blood pressure; → pulse rate	Cardioselective agents may also inhibit β₂-receptors in higher doses (eg, all may aggravate asthma)
Betaxolol† (Kerlone)	5-20	1/day		
Bisoprolol† (Zebeta)	2.5-10	1/day		
Metoprolol† (Lopressor)	50-100	1 or 2/day		
Metoprolol XR† (Toprol-XL)	50-100	1/day		
Nadolol (Corgard)	40-120	1/day		
Propranolol LA (Inderal LA)	60-180	1/day		
Propranolol XL (InnoPran XL)	80-120	1/day (night)		
Timolol (Blocadren)	20-40	1/day		

β-Blockers With ISA[‡]			
Acebutolol[†] (Sectral)	200-800	2/day	Possible advantage in subjects with bradycardia who require a β-blocker—they may produce fewer metabolic effects
Penbutolol (Levatol)	10-40	1/day	Less effect on heart rate and vascular and bronchial smooth muscle
Pindolol (Generic)	10-40	2/day	

Abbreviation: LA, long acting; XR, extended release.

* Dosages may also differ from the manufacturer's prescribing information recommendations. These dosages are based on our experience and the belief that if small or moderate doses of one drug prove ineffective, small doses of a medication from another class should be added.

† Cardioselective.

‡ ISA = intrinsic sympathomimetic action (slight β$_2$-receptor stimulation).

6

- These agents are more slowly metabolized and are excreted through the kidney
- Their duration of action is longer
- There may be fewer CNS side effects.

This, however, is also not invariable. In our experience, most of the β-blockers (including those with ISA) in appropriate doses reduce BP to an equal degree, so that choice between the various agents depends upon:
- Side effects
- Duration of action
- Tolerability.

β-Blockers appear to be:
- Especially effective in young, white hypertensive patients
- Especially effective in patients with resting tachycardia
- Preferentially indicated in hypertensive patients with angina or a previous myocardial infarction (MI)
- Useful as add-on therapy (in addition to an angiotensin-converting enzyme [ACE] inhibitor, diuretic, and digitalis) in congestive heart failure (CHF) regardless of whether the patient is hypertensive.

β-Adrenergic receptor blockers have been used either as second-step therapy in many of the clinical trials or as alternative first-step drugs to diuretics in the Heart Attack Primary Prevention in Hypertension (HAPPHY), Metoprolol Atherosclerosis Prevention in Hypertension (MAPHY), Medical Research Council (MRC) in Older Patients, and the Swedish Trials in Old Patients With Hypertension (STOP-Hypertension and STOP-Hypertension-2) studies. In only one of the large trials have β-blockers been found to reduce the incidence of a first MI to a greater degree than diuretics (MAPHY). This study was actually an extension of another trial; interpretation of the results has been questioned. In the MRC in the elderly trial, a β-blocker proved less effective than a diuretic in preventing CHD mortality, but results are also difficult to interpret because of the high dropout rate in the treatment groups. The STOP-Hypertension-2 trial demonstrated that a β-blocker/diuretic–treated group achieved the same overall mortality/morbidity results as a group treated with an ACE inhibitor/calcium channel blocker (CCB).

In general, the use of β-blockers in elderly subjects reduces BP to goal levels in fewer subjects than the use of diuretics. This may account for the fact that they may be less effective in reducing CHD events in elderly hypertensives. Stroke and heart failure are, however, reduced significantly in this population when β-blockers are given. β-Adrenergic inhibitors have been shown to prevent a second MI in patients with known ischemic heart disease and to reduce overall mortality in both high- and low-risk patients (**Table 6.2**).

A meta-analysis of the available data with β-blockers, primarily propranolol and timolol, suggests a reduction of 20% to 33% in infarctions and overall mortality. These positive results with β-blockers in post-MI patients are considerably better than outcome data on the CCBs, where consistent evidence for reduction in events in patients with ischemic heart disease is lacking. Data with two of the β-blockers, bisoprolol (Zebeta) and metoprolol (Toprol-XL), indicate a decrease in cardiovascular (CV) events and all-cause mortality in patients with preexisting heart failure when these agents are added to treatment in patients who were already receiving standard therapy with an ACE inhibitor and a diuretic. These latter studies have been helpful in dispelling the perception that β-blockers are contraindicated in patients with CHF. As noted, recent data from the United Kingdom Prospective Diabetes Study

TABLE 6.2 — RESULTS OF β-BLOCKER TRIALS ON MORBIDITY AND MORTALITY IN PATIENTS POST–MYOCARDIAL INFARCTION
Number of Patients Randomized • Controls .... 9334 • Treated 9721
Reduction in Risk-Treated Compared With Controls • Sudden death .... 33% • Nonfatal infarctions .... 20% • Overall mortality .... 22% • Nonsudden death 20%
Results are all highly significant.

(UKPDS) with a β-blocker–based treatment program in type 2 diabetes indicate a similar decrease in CV events as an ACE inhibitor–based program in patients with good BP control. These results should help to dispel the perception that β-blockers should not be used in diabetics. Results of the study in hypertensive African American patients with kidney disease and proteinuria (African American Study of Kidney Disease [AASK]) indicate that a β-blocker (metoprolol) may be somewhat more effective in preventing progression of renal disease than a CCB (amlodipine) but less effective than an ACE inhibitor.

Side Effects

In general, β-adrenergic inhibitors are well tolerated, but some patients develop annoying side effects, especially when these agents are used in large doses (**Table 6.3**).

■ Pulmonary

Noncardioselective β-blockers may produce symptomatic shortness of breath or asthma in patients who are susceptible to a decrease in air flow. These findings are not common, but they occur often enough to warrant a statement that these agents should not be used or only used with care in a patient with asthma or chronic obstructive pulmonary disease. Cardio-selective β-blockers such as bisoprolol and atenolol may decrease air movement to a somewhat lesser degree. A history of asthma, however, should still be considered a relative contraindication to the use of any β-adrenergic inhibitor.

■ **Cardiac**
- *Bradycardia*—It is probably not a good idea to use β-adrenergic inhibitors as initial therapy in patients with resting heart rates of <50 to 55.
- *Fatigue*—The decrease in cardiac output and flow to peripheral muscle groups may result in feelings of fatigue. This is probably the most annoying side effect of the β-blockers, especially in people who are accustomed to vigorous exercise and in some older people. Lower doses may reduce the possibility of this effect.
- *Decrease in the rate of atrioventricular conduction*—This may worsen heart block. β-Blockers should not be used in patients with greater than first-degree heart block.
- *Central effects*—The type of fatigue seen in some patients on β-blockers may be related to a decrease in cardiac output; in other cases, it may be secondary to a central effect. Nightmares, insomnia, or vivid dreams may be noted. These can be disturbing. Although some studies have suggested that depression is a common side effect with β-adrenergic inhibitors, this is not true in our experience, at least in the dosages prescribed. There is some evidence that CNS effects are less common with the less lipid-soluble β-blockers (eg, atenolol or nadolol compared with propranolol).

TABLE 6.3 — SIDE EFFECTS OF β-ADRENERGIC INHIBITORS

Symptoms/Signs	Cautions	Comments
Bradycardia*	Should not be used in patients (a) with heart rate <50, (b) with more than first-degree heart block, or (c) with sick sinus syndrome	Usually not a problem in most people
Fatigue	May indicate adverse effect on cardiac output, central effect, or as a result of ↓ in peripheral muscle blood flow	Some limitation of exercise tolerance (may be a problem); use smaller doses
Insomnia, bizarre dreams, or nightmares	May represent first signs of depression (which does occur in a small number of patients on a β-blocker)	May be less common with cardio-selective agents
Cold hands, exacerbation of Raynaud's phenomenon, or increase in symptoms of peripheral arterial disease*	Avoid, if possible, in subjects with definite evidence of peripheral vascular disease or Raynaud's phenomenon	Using small doses or agents with intrinsic sympathomimetic activity (ISA) may reduce this symptom

Sexual dysfunction	May cause impotence/loss of libido—men; loss of libido/delayed orgasm—women	May occur in approximately 5% of patients
Dyspnea, flare-up of asthma	Avoid or use with great care in patients with chronic obstructive pulmonary disease or a history of asthma	Unusual in patients without pulmonary disease
Metabolic Changes		
↑ Triglycerides, ↓ HDL levels*	Monitor lipids; if definite change occurs, consider other drugs if possible	Clinical significance of questionable importance
Mask symptoms and signs of hypoglycemia	Probably avoid use in insulin-dependent diabetics	Tremor and tachycardia inhibited in insulin shock (sweating intact); recovery delayed
* Less with β-blockers with ISA.		

* Less with β-blockers with ISA.

In several comparative studies of β-blockers, diuretics, and ACE inhibitors, there were no differences observed in quality-of-life measurements among these drugs (except for propranolol, where quality of life was diminished). In a comparative placebo-controlled study (Treatment of Mild Hypertension Study [TOMHS]) of five different classes of drugs, β-blockers and diuretics were both found to improve quality-of-life measurements compared with several other medications.

Metabolic Changes Secondary to β-Blockers

- A long-term increase in triglyceride levels and a slight decrease in high-density lipoprotein (HDL) levels have been noted in patients taking β-blockers without ISA. This effect is less for β-blockers with ISA. The clinical significance of these changes has not been determined. As noted, these drugs reduce recurrence of MI and mortality in patients with ischemic heart disease.

- In patients taking a β-blocker, prolonged hypoglycemia may occur in insulin-dependent diabetics who experience an insulin reaction. This phenomenon may actually be seen more commonly in the future in view of recent data suggesting that rigid control of blood glucose levels will reduce CV risk. More careful control may lead to more frequent insulin reactions; these may be aggravated in some patients taking a β-blocker.

- A β-blocker may mask symptoms of insulin-induced hypoglycemia. Tremor and tachycardia associated with catecholamine release may be blunted or eliminated by β-adrenergic inhibitors. Sweating, however, is not decreased by the use of these agents. These facts must be considered in any patient on a β-blocker who arrives in the emergency room in coma or semi-coma with bradycardia and lacking the usual symptoms of an insulin reaction.

Changes in Renal Blood Flow

In some patients taking β-blockers, there is a decrease in renal blood flow, reflecting possible renal vessel constriction. This may not be of great clinical significance and has not been reported with atenolol or nadolol.

6

Place in Therapy

β-Blockers have been recommended as one of the alternative medications for initial therapy in the management of hypertension. Most people tolerate them well, and when β-blockers are used as monotherapy, about 40% to 50% of patients will respond. Compared with the response to diuretics or CCBs, BP response to a β-blocker is less in black patients and there is evidence that the elderly may not respond as well as younger patients.

In combination with small doses of a diuretic, however, these agents are highly effective in all patient groups. The Food and Drug Administration has approved bisoprolol (2.5, 5.0, or 10 mg)/hydrochlorothiazide (HCTZ) (6.25 mg) combination (Ziac) as initial therapy. While a 6.25-mg dose of HCTZ is effective in only a small percentage of subjects as monotherapy, the number of responders increases significantly when it is combined with the β-blocker. There are other effective combinations of β-blockers and diuretics available (eg, Corzide, Lopressor HCT, Tenoretic) (**Table 5.6**). BP is lowered to goal levels in about 75% to 80% of patients with this type of combination therapy.

The Sixth Joint National Committee (JNC-VI) on Prevention, Detection, Evaluation, and Treatment of High Blood Pressure in 1997 had suggested that in elderly patients "*thiazide diuretics or β-blockers in combination with thiazide diuretics are recommended because they are effective in reducing mortality and morbidity in older persons with hypertension as shown in multiple randomized controlled trials.*" JNC 7 indicates special situations for the use of β-blockers and that a β-blocker/diuretic combination may be one of the choices for initial or first-step therapy in the management of stage 2 hypertension (BP >160/100 mm Hg) or in patients with hypertension and evidence of CHD. A β-blocker should be used in almost every post-MI patient unless there is a contraindication to its use (eg, pulmonary symptoms, marked bradycardia or heart block, or severe peripheral vascular disease). Based on data for several β-blockers (bisoprolol, metoprolol), the use of these agents in patients with heart failure may reduce CV events, sudden cardiac death, and all-cause mortality.

As mentioned, data from the 8.4-year comparative UKPDS indicate the effectiveness of a β-blocker–based treatment program in reducing CV events in type 2 diabetics if BP is carefully controlled, which should reduce some concerns that physicians have had about using a β-blocker in type 2 diabetics.

β-Blockers may not be *the* drugs of choice in hypertensive diabetics but obviously they can be used safely with the expectation that a reduction in CV events will be noted if BP is reduced.

7 Combined α_1- and β-Blockers

Two combinations of an α_1-blocker plus a β-blocker are approved in the United States for use in patients with hypertension (**Table 7.1**):

- Labetalol (Normodyne, Trandate), which combines a nonspecific β_1- and β_2-blocker with some α_1-blocking activity
- Carvedilol (Coreg), a β-blocker with vasodilatory properties secondary to α_1-blocking activity.

These agents possess a greater degree of β-adrenergic inhibiting activity than α_1-blocking activity. Blood pressure (BP) is reduced, mainly as a result of a decrease in peripheral resistance. There is less effect on heart rate and cardiac output than with the β-adrenergic inhibitors alone. Heart rate decreases only to a slight degree; in addition, there is less fluid retention and orthostatic hypotension than with α_1-blockers alone. Changes in renin and catecholamine levels are minimal (**Table 7.2**).

Labetalol and carvedilol are effective antihypertensive agents. Two of the more common side effects of these drugs are postural hypotension and dizziness, which are noted in between 8% and 10% of patients. These side effects occur not only on initial dosing, but may be noted with increasing dose levels. Fatigue, headache, and tingling of the scalp have been reported in about 5% of patients. Titration to an effective dose may be time-consuming, especially with labetalol. This drug has a short duration of action and multiple daily doses may be necessary. For these reasons, labetalol

TABLE 7.1 — COMBINED α_1- AND β-BLOCKERS USED IN THE TREATMENT OF HYPERTENSION

Generic (Trade) Name	Usual Dosage Range		Physiologic Effects	Comments
	Dose (mg)	Frequency		
Carvedilol (Coreg)	6.25-25	2/day	Cardiac output and renal blood flow maintained, blood pressure decreased, *antioxidant effects*	Beneficial effects in heart failure; may decrease myocardial damage post–myocardial infarction
Labetalol (Normodyne, Trandate)	200-800	2/day	Cardiac output $\pm \downarrow$, $\downarrow$ plasma renin activity, $\downarrow$ blood pressure, some decrease in pulse rate	Probably more effective in blacks than other β-blockers; may cause postural effects; titration should be based on standing blood pressures

has not been widely accepted in the United States as a suitable initial treatment agent. The Seventh Joint National Committee on Prevention, Detection, Evaluation, and Treatment of High Blood Pressure has recommended this class of medications as possible add-on therapy or in patients with specific or compelling indications.

Part of the problem with labetalol may have been the high dosages that were originally advocated. If a dosage of only 100 mg twice a day is used initially, with an increase to a maximum of only 400 to 500 mg/day, side effects are less frequent (when the drug was introduced, doses of up to 1200 mg/day were commonly prescribed).

One adverse reaction that is noted with β-blockers is hair loss; this may be less frequent with labetalol. As with other agents, if small doses of a drug in this class are ineffective, combining it with a small dose of a diuretic increases response significantly.

Carvedilol, the newer α_1–β-blocker:

- Has a longer duration of action than labetalol
- In our experience, is usually effective in a once-a-day dose; and

- Is relatively simple to titrate in the management of hypertension (this may be more difficult in patients with heart failure).

Labetalol and carvedilol are effective in black patients to a greater degree than β-blockers, and they lower BP to the same degree as a β-blocker and an α_1-blocker given as separate medications. Intravenous labetalol has been shown to be useful in the treatment of hypertensive crises or accelerated hypertension. Labetalol or carvedilol can be used as alternative initial monotherapy in the management of hypertension but should be prescribed with caution in the elderly. *Titration of a drug for BP-lowering effects in this population should be based on levels of standing BP.*

Carvedilol has been extensively tested in patients with congestive heart failure who remained symptomatic on an angiotensin-converting enzyme (ACE) inhibitor, a diuretic, and digitalis. Results indicate a definite reduction in morbidity and mortality when this drug is given over and above that achieved with previous "triple-drug therapy." Animal and human studies indicate that carvedilol has antioxidant properties considerably greater than vitamin E, in addition to its β- and α_1-blocking properties. Oxidation of low-density lipoprotein (LDL), an essential element in the atherogenic process, is reduced. This may account for the beneficial effects of reducing the degree of myocardial muscle damage in experimental myocardial infarction. This effect and effects on cell proliferation may also be responsible for preventing or delaying the atherogenic process in animal models.

Additional experiences with this agent over the past 2 years continue to validate benefits in patients with heart failure. The antioxidant properties of carvedilol may present some unique advantages in the treatment of hypertensive patients and patients with ischemic heart disease.

8 Peripheral Adrenergic Inhibitors

The drugs in this class are used infrequently, primarily because numerous other medications are now available that are better tolerated. Two of them, guanethidine (Ismelin) and guanadrel (Hylorel), are highly potent medications and inhibit the activity of the sympathetic nervous system by blocking the exit of norepinephrine from storage granules.

Guanethidine was widely used in the 1950s and 1960s. It is effective on a once-a-day basis even in severe hypertension, and when combined with a diuretic, reduces blood pressure (BP) in a high percentage of patients. The occurrence of severe postural hypotension, diarrhea, and sexual dysfunction in some patients greatly limits its usefulness. Guanethidine in small doses of 10 to 20 mg/day in combination with a diuretic may prove effective in a few patients who are resistant to other therapy. Unlike some other antihypertensive agents, increasing the dose of guanethidine increases the degree of BP reduction. The dose-response curve is not as flat as with other medications. Its use must be monitored carefully.

Guanadrel is similar to guanethidine but has a shorter duration of action.

Reserpine acts on the central nervous system by decreasing the transport of norepinephrine into storage granules; eventually the amount of norepinephrine available when nerves are stimulated is reduced. This drug has been in use in the United States since the early 1950s. When reserpine is given in combination with a diuretic, BP is reduced to goal levels of <140/90 mm

Hg in about 70% to 75% of patients, a degree of response similar to that noted with other combinations.

Unfortunately, when reserpine or its derivatives were used in the 1950s and early 1960s, doses that were unnecessarily high (eg, ≥0.5 to 1 mg/day) were given. Side effects, including nasal stuffiness, sedation, and most important, depression, were not uncommon. But in those early days of antihypertensive drug treatment, many of us thought that the higher the dose, the better the response, with any of the BP-lowering agents. This included the β-blockers (propranolol was given in doses of up to 3 g/day), hydralazine (often given in doses up to 1200 mg/day), α-methyldopa (up to 2 to 3 g/day), and even diuretics (eg, up to the equivalent of 200 mg/day of chlorthalidone).

Today, we know that most of these drugs are effective at much smaller doses. In fact, as repeatedly mentioned, they have a relatively flat dose-response curve. Reserpine in small doses of 0.05 to 0.1 mg *in combination with a diuretic* is effective (**Table 5**.6) and has the advantage of being inexpensive; most patients tolerate it well at these dose levels. Physicians should be on the alert, however, for the occasional patient who develops symptoms of depression, such as:

- Fatigue
- Insomnia
- Dreams
- General lack of interest in daily activities, job, etc.

Symptoms may persist for many weeks after the drug is discontinued.

Combinations of diuretics with reserpine (Hydropres, Diupres) or the whole-root rauwolfia (Rauzide) are available but may be difficult to obtain (**Table 5**.6). **Table 8**.1 lists dosages and side effects of peripheral adrenergic inhibitors. As with other tables in this book, maximum suggested doses may be lower than those given in the manufacturer's prescribing information.

TABLE 8.1 — PERIPHERAL-ACTING ADRENERGIC INHIBITORS*

Generic (Trade) Name	Usual Dosage Range Dose (mg)	Usual Dosage Range Frequency	Adverse Reactions	Physiologic Effects	Comments
Guanadrel (Hylorel)*	10-20	2/day	Sexual dysfunction, dizziness, diarrhea	Inhibits catecholamine release from neuronal storage sites	May cause orthostatic and exercise-induced hypotension
Guanethidine (Ismelin)*	10-20	1/day			
Rauwolfia Alkaloids					
Rauwolfia serpentina*	50-100	1/day	Depression, nasal stuffiness, activation of peptic ulcer	Depletion of tissue stores of catecholamines	Depression may persist for weeks following discontinuation of drug
Reserpine					
Reserpine*	0.05-0.1	1/day			
Reserpine combinations	See Table 5.6	1/day			

* These agents are used infrequently, but may be helpful in some cases, especially when used in combination with a diuretic.

8

This modification is based on long experience and on the fact that most of these drugs are used in combination with a diuretic. While the current emphasis on the use of small doses of two different types of antihypertensive medications rather than large doses of one type may appear to represent a new approach, it is not. Reserpine combinations were in common use in the 1960s.

9   Central Agonists

The central agonists are also used infrequently. They have an unusual mechanism of action in the vasomotor centers of the brain. By stimulating central α_2-receptors, they increase inhibitory neuron activity and decrease sympathetic outflow from the central nervous system. Their hemodynamic effects include:

- A decrease in peripheral resistance
- A slight decrease in cardiac output
- A decrease in blood pressure (BP).

Among the available central agonists are:

- α-Methyldopa (Aldomet)
- Clonidine (Catapres)
- Guanfacine (Tenex).

These medications reduce BP to normotensive levels in about 35% to 50% of patients, and in combination with small doses of a diuretic, are even more effective.

But side effects occur in a high percentage of patients and dropout rates from therapy can be as high as 20% to 30%. In addition, studies have shown that quality-of-life measurements are decreased more when these drugs are used than when diuretics, angiotensin-converting enzyme (ACE) inhibitors, most β-blockers, or calcium channel blockers (CCBs) are given. **Table 9.**1 lists these agents, along with their physiologic effects and adverse reactions. The most common side effects include:

- Sedation
- Dry mouth
- Drowsiness

TABLE 9.1 — CENTRAL AGONISTS USED FOR TREATING HYPERTENSION

Generic (Trade) Name	Usual Dosage Range		Adverse Reactions	Physiologic Effects	Comments
	Dose (mg)	Frequency			
Clonidine (Catapres)	0.1-0.8	2/day	Dry mouth, drowsiness, headache, fatigue, depression	Stimulate central α_2-receptors that inhibit efferent sympathetic activity—blood pressure ↓; peripheral resistance ↓; no significant effect on heart rate, CO, renal blood flow or GFR	Clonidine patch is replaced once a week. None of these agents should be withdrawn abruptly because of rebound hypertension
Clonidine patch (Catapres-TTS)	0.1-0.3	1/week			
Guanfacine (Generic)	0.5-2	1/day			
Methyldopa (Aldomet)	250-1000	2/day	Possible immune reactions		
Reserpine (Generic)	0.05-0.25	1/day			

Abbreviations: CO, cardiac output; GFR, glomerular filtration rate.

- Dizziness
- Fatigue
- Headache
- Depression
- Dreams.

Symptoms of depression may be subtle, as they are with reserpine, and include a decrease in mental alertness, vivid dreams, or a decrease in the ability to enjoy life.

In addition to the above adverse effects, which are shared by methyldopa, clonidine, guanabenz, and guanfacine, methyldopa may induce certain auto-immune disorders. Abnormal liver function tests and fever may occur in 5% to 10% of patients, and a positive Coombs' test in as many as 35% to 40%. Hemolytic anemia, however, is uncommon.

Doses of methyldopa should probably not exceed 750 to 1000 mg/day. Doses closer to the starting range (ie, 250 mg/day) should be used in combination with a diuretic when this drug is used.

Clonidine is similar in action to α-methyldopa, with a somewhat shorter duration of action when given orally. It can be absorbed through the skin and is available as a transdermal patch; duration of action is increased considerably. The 0.1-mg patch should be changed every 7 days. Local skin reactions occur in as many as 30% of patients with the transdermal patch. When used orally, the initial dosage of clonidine should be 0.1 mg twice a day, increasing to a maximum dosage of 0.3 or 0.4 mg twice a day. Small doses of a diuretic should probably be used with clonidine to increase effectiveness and reduce side effects rather than increase the dosage to higher levels.

Drowsiness, dry mouth, and fatigue are the most common side effects with clonidine therapy. Use of the patch may result in fewer adverse reactions. A deterrent to the widespread use of clonidine is the fact that if the drug is stopped, the sympathetic nervous system becomes overactive from a suppressed state; there can be a marked overshoot in BP with episodes of severe hypertension. This diagnosis should be considered in any patient who abruptly stops clonidine therapy; restarting the drug will reduce BP. The clonidine patch has also been used in the treatment of nicotine addiction with varying results.

Guanabenz is similar to clonidine. Starting dosages are about 2 mg to 4 mg twice a day; the maximum dose should probably not exceed 16 mg/day. Guanfacine is similar, with a dose range of 1 to 3 mg/day (**Table 9.1**).

The use of this class of drugs has decreased in recent years because of the availability of medications that are better tolerated. However, some possible indications for central agonists are:

- Insulin-dependent diabetics who are resistent to therapy with an ACE inhibitor or angiotensin II receptor blocker (ARB) and a diuretic
- Patients with asthma or those with peripheral arterial disease who do not respond to a diuretic, CCB, ACE inhibitor, or ARB and in whom a β-blocker should probably not be used
- In patients who have experienced annoying side effects with ACE inhibitors (angioedema, cough) or CCBs (palpitations, dizziness, persistent edema, constipation)
- As a third- or fourth-step medication in patients who have not responded to other drugs—the "resistant" hypertensive.

Methyldopa is still used in treating the hypertension of toxemia of pregnancy. Details of management of this entity can be found in any standard textbook on hypertension.

10 α_1-Adrenergic Inhibitors

Currently, there are three selective α_1-blockers available in the United States:

- Doxazosin (Cardura)
- Prazosin (Minipress)
- Terazosin (Hytrin).

These drugs act by blocking or inhibiting the postsynaptic α_1-receptors on vascular smooth muscle. This inhibits the uptake of catecholamines by smooth muscle cells. Vasoconstriction is blunted, and peripheral vasodilation occurs (**Figure 10**.1).

There are also several *nonselective* α-blockers available, ie, phentolamine (Regitine) and phenoxybenzamine (Dibenzyline). These agents block not only the postsynaptic α_1-receptors, but also the presynaptic α_2-receptors located on the neuronal membrane itself. These drugs have not proved effective for the long-term management of hypertension. Although they reduce blood pressure (BP) (often dramatically), their action on α_2-receptors removes an inhibiting effect on norepinephrine release; more of this substance is released into the circulation, tachycardia occurs, and tachyphylaxis to BP lowering follows fairly quickly. In addition, postural hypotension and other adverse reactions mitigate against the use of these agents, except in the therapy for pheochromocytoma, for which they are highly effective.

Although it has been shown that the α_1-receptor blockers (ie, doxazosin, prazosin, and terazosin) reduce diastolic blood pressure (DBP) to as great an extent as other classes of antihypertensive drugs, our experience suggests that their effect on systolic BP is

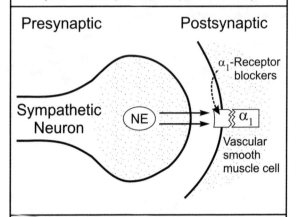

**FIGURE 10.1 — MODE OF
ACTION OF α_1-BLOCKERS
(DOXAZOSIN, PRAZOSIN, TERAZOSIN)**

Presynaptic   Postsynaptic

α_1-Receptor
blockers

Sympathetic
Neuron   NE α_1

Vascular
smooth
muscle cell

Abbreviation: NE, norepinephrine.

A schematic representation of a neuron and a vascular
smooth muscle cell showing how α_1-blockers block the
α_1-receptor.

Adapted from: *Clinical Hypertension*. 5th ed. Baltimore, Md:
Williams & Wilkins; 1990:211.

somewhat less. In addition, symptomatic side effects
occur in a higher percentage of patients than with some
of the other drugs. For example, in a 1-year study of
an α_1-receptor blocker (prazosin), 18 of 42 patients
dropped out of therapy because of adverse reactions.
In a comparative study, only three patients out of 48
on hydrochlorothiazide discontinued therapy. Side effects of α_1-receptor blockers include:

- Postural hypotension
- Tachycardia
- Dizziness
- Occasional gastrointestinal distress.

Postural hypotension and dizziness may occur with initiation of therapy or with any increase in dosage. These side effects are less common with the longer-acting α_1-blocker doxazosin (Cardura). Dosage should be started at 1 mg/day at bedtime. There is little reason, in our opinion, to use >2 mg bid of these agents except in unusual circumstances. An α_1-blocker, such as doxazosin (Cardura), can be used as a third-step drug in combination with a diuretic and a β-adrenergic inhibitor. Dosages are kept to a minimum, which results in fewer and more tolerable side effects. These medications are effective in reducing DBP if it has not been brought to normotensive levels with other medications. We have rarely used any of these agents as initial monotherapy; in view of recent data (see below), this decision is a reasonable one. **Table 10**.1 reviews actions, side effects, and dosages of α_1-receptor blockers.

Several trials have demonstrated that α_1-receptor blockers may have a favorable effect on lipid levels. In comparative studies with four other medications, doxazosin was shown to decrease cholesterol levels and raise high-density lipoprotein (HDL) levels to a greater degree than other agents. In addition, there is some evidence that these drugs will reduce plasma insulin levels and improve glucose tolerance (not all studies have confirmed this). Because of these possible advantages, it has been suggested that the α_1-blockers may be ideal antihypertensive agents. However, because symptomatic adverse reactions may be fairly common, α_1-blockers have not been widely accepted by physicians as step-1 therapy. The α_1-blockers have a favorable effect on symptoms of prostatic hypertrophy and are recommended in small doses in the management of older hypertensive men with this problem. Other agents should be used, if necessary, to maintain goal BP levels.

Recent data from the randomized, blinded Antihypertensive and Lipid-Lowering Treatment to Prevent

TABLE 10.1 — α₁-RECEPTOR BLOCKERS USED TO TREAT HYPERTENSION

Generic (Trade) Name	Usual Dosage Range		Adverse Reactions	Physiologic Effects	Comments
	Dose (mg)	Frequency			
Doxazosin (Cardura)	1-16	1/day	Dizziness, palpitations, GI disturbances	Block postsynaptic α_1-receptors vasodilation—peripheral resistance $\downarrow$; BP $\downarrow$	All may cause postural effects; titration should be based on standing BP
Prazosin (Minipress)	2-20	2 or 3/day			
Terazosin (Hytrin)	1-20	1-2/day			

Abbreviations: BP, blood pressure; GI, gastrointestinal.

Heart Attack Trial (ALLHAT) indicate that the use of doxazosin resulted in a doubling of the incidence of heart failure and an increase in angina and myocardial infarction when compared with a diuretic. The use of the α-blocker was discontinued in this study and recommendations that these are not preferred initial therapy agents in the management of hypertension followed the release of these findings.

10

11   Direct Vasodilators

Two vasodilators, hydralazine (Apresoline) and minoxidil (Loniten) have been available for the treatment of hypertension for many years. They act directly on vascular smooth muscle (as potassium channel openers?). Hydralazine was used for many years in combination with reserpine and a diuretic; later, in the 1950s and 1960s, it was used as a third-step drug with a β-blocker and a diuretic. These combinations effectively lowered blood pressure (BP) in a high percentage of patients, even those with severe hypertension. Diastolic BP is often reduced more effectively when hydralazine is added to other drugs.

As a result of dilation of arterioles with a decrease in peripheral resistance and BP, baroreceptors are stimulated; an increase in heart rate and release of catecholamines results (**Table 11.1**). This may lead to renal retention of sodium with expansion of fluid volume. Because of these effects, hydralazine or minoxidil alone may be only temporarily effective as a BP-lowering agent. Tachyphylaxis to their effects develops rapidly. Side effects such as the following also limit their usefulness as monotherapeutic agents:

- Tachycardia
- Fluid retention
- Flushing
- Headache
- In the case of minoxidil, excessive hair growth, not just on the face but on the body. This is especially troublesome in women, and the drug should probably not be used in women except in the rare case of severe hypertension that is resistant to multiple-drug therapy (eg, renal insufficiency).

TABLE 11.1 — DIRECT VASODILATORS USED IN TREATING HYPERTENSION

Generic (Trade) Name	Usual Dosage Range		Adverse Reactions	Physiologic Effects	Comments
	Dose (mg)	Frequency			
Hydralazine (Apresoline)	25-100	2/day	Tachycardia, flushing, headache, fluid retention, lupuslike reaction	Direct smooth muscle vasodilation (primarily arteriolar)	Subject to phenotypically determined metabolism (acetylation)
Minoxidil (Loniten)	2.5-4-80	1 or 2/day	Tachycardia, flushing, headache, fluid retention, excessive hair growth	See hydralazine	Both agents: should use with a diuretic and β-blocker to minimize fluid retention and reflex tachycardia

The compensatory mechanism that prevents long-term BP lowering and produces side effects may be mitigated by the concurrent use of an adrenergic inhibitor (ie, reserpine) or a β-blocker. In patients on minoxidil, large doses of a potent diuretic may have to be used to prevent the massive accumulation of fluid that may occur. In these cases, drugs such as furosemide (Lasix) may be needed in doses of up to ≥200 mg/day, metolazone (Zaroxolyn or Diulo) in doses of up to 10 mg/day, or torsemide (Demadex) in doses of up to 15 to 20 mg a day.

Hydralazine is prescribed very infrequently and usually only as a third drug if BP is not controlled by a diuretic plus a β-blocker, an angiotensin-converting enzymne (ACE) inhibitor, or an angiotensin II receptor blocker (ARB). In some patients who do not respond to a diuretic plus a β-blocker, hydralazine may be useful in an approximate starting dosage of 25 mg twice a day, increasing to about 100 mg to 150 mg twice a day. Dosages higher than these should probably not be used because a lupuslike syndrome may occur at higher doses. This is not common, but positive antinuclear antibody (ANA) tests may occur in as many as 40% of patients. If a patient who is taking hydralazine does develop a fever, rash, or arthralgias, the drug should be discontinued and other drugs substituted.

Minoxidil is rarely, if ever, used as initial therapy and its use is limited to patients with severe hypertension and renal insufficiency, or to patients resistant to or unable to tolerate other medications. As noted, fluid retention and hirsutism are the most commonly noted side effects.

Although direct vasodilators are effective antihypertensive drugs, there is little or no place for them as initial monotherapy, and other drugs that reduce peripheral resistance have largely taken their place, ie, ACE inhibitors, ARBs, or calcium channel blockers. Hydralazine is useful in some cases of accelerated or malig-

145

nant hypertension or in toxemia of pregnancy. **Table 11.2** lists possible indications for the use of this drug.

TABLE 11.2 — WHEN TO USE HYDRALAZINE (APRESOLINE)

- In patients with or without renal insufficiency, if blood pressure is not normalized by a diuretic plus a β-blocker, ACE inhibitor, CCB, ARB, or a diuretic plus reserpine
- As part of therapy for malignant or accelerated hypertension when there is a reason not to use a CCB, an ACE inhibitor, or an ARB
- Intravenously in a hypertensive crisis or preeclampsia

Abbreviations: ACE, angiotensin-converting enzyme; ARB, angiotensin II receptor blocker; CCB, calcium channel blocker.

---

12 ACE Inhibitors

Angiotensin-converting enzyme (ACE) inhibitors are among the most effective vasodilating antihypertensive drugs. These drugs prevent the conversion of angiotensin I, an inactive octapeptide, to angiotensin II, which is a potent vasoconstrictor and aldosterone stimulator (**Figure 12**.1). In addition, ACE inhibitors prevent the degradation of bradykinin (a vasodilator substance) by inhibiting kininase II, an enzyme that inactivates bradykinin. Bradykinin levels are increased, enhancing the synthesis of various prostaglandins (which also act as vasodilators). *Thus ACE inhibitors have a combined action of decreasing the generation of angiotensin II and increasing the levels of bradykinin and various vasodilating prostaglandins.*

ACE inhibitors are effective as monotherapy. In studies comparing different classes of drugs, blood pressure (BP) reduction with ACE inhibitors is essentially equivalent to that with the other medications, except in black patients who are less responsive. A list of ACE inhibitors currently available in the United States is given in **Table 12**.1. Others are under investigation. Most ACE inhibitors have similar actions although they differ chemically. Some contain a sulfhydryl group (ie, captopril). This may be a factor in causing some of this drug's side effects, such as loss of taste; however, this has not been proven.

ACE inhibitors differ in duration of action and mode of excretion and, therefore, in frequency of administration (**Table 12**.1). They produce some degree of natriuresis and potassium retention as a result of decreasing aldosterone secretion. BP decreases because of vasodilation and reduction in peripheral resistance. Cardiac output is not decreased, and despite the de-

FIGURE 12.1—SITE OF ACTION OF ACE INHIBITORS AND ANGIOTENSIN II RECEPTOR BLOCKERS

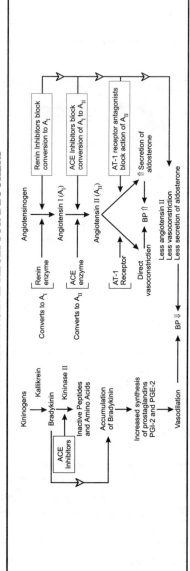

I. Mode of action of angiotensin-converting enzyme (ACE) inhibitors: block conversion of A_I (an inactive substance) to A_{II} (a vasoconstrictor). This action (1) decreases the generation of A_{II}, and also by blocking the activity of kininase II, (2) decreases the breakdown of bradykinin: this vasodilator substance increases; blood pressure is lowered.

II. Mode of action of *angiotensin II (AT-1) receptor blocker:* blocks effects of A_{II} peripherally; aldosterone secretion is not increased and vasoconstriction is prevented; *no effect on bradykinin system.* Does not prevent production of angiotensin II.

148

TABLE 12.1 — ACE INHIBITORS USED FOR TREATING HYPERTENSION

Generic (Trade) Name	Usual Dosage Range		Adverse Reactions	Physiologic Effects	Comments
	Dose (mg)	Frequency			
Benazepril (Lotensin)	10-40	1 or 2/day	*Cough*, rash, loss of taste, palpitations, rarely angioedema	Blocks formation of angiotensin II, promoting vasodilation and decreased aldosterone; also increases bradykinin and vasodilator prostaglandins	Diuretic doses should be reduced before starting angiotensin-converting enzyme (ACE) inhibitor whenever possible to prevent excessive hypotension. Smaller doses in patients with serum creatinine >3.0 mg/dL. May cause hyperkalemia in patients with renal impairment or in those receiving potassium-sparing agents. Can cause renal failure in patients with bilateral renal artery stenosis
Captopril (Capoten)	25-100	2/day			
Enalapril (Vasotec)	2.5-40	1 or 2/day			
Fosinopril (Monopril)	10-40	1/day			
Lisinopril (Zestril, Prinivil)	10-40	1/day			
Moexipril (Univasc)	7.5-30	1/day			
Perindopril (Aceon)	4-8	1 or 2/day			
Quinapril (Accupril)	10-40	1/day			
Ramipril (Altace)	2.5-20	1/day			
Trandolapril (Mavik)	1-4	1/day			

12

crease in BP, there is usually only a slight increase in heart rate. We have, however, seen some patients who develop a persistent low-grade tachycardia following the use of an ACE inhibitor.

In addition to their effect on elevated BP, the ACE inhibitors are particularly effective as unloading agents in the treatment of heart failure because of the reduction in afterload. In heart failure, levels of angiotensin II are high; reducing these levels or blocking the activity of this pressor substance is beneficial and may have a favorable effect on cardiac function over and above the effect on vascular resistance. In long-term studies, patients with heart failure have improved in exercise tolerance and other symptoms following the addition of an ACE inhibitor to standard therapy with digitalis and diuretics. In addition, morbidity and mortality have been reduced. Mortality from recurrent myocardial infarction (MI) has also been reduced by the use of ACE inhibitors in patients with ischemic heart disease and reduced left ventricular function (ejection fractions <40%).

ACE inhibitors are one of the groups of drugs suggested as first-step therapy by the 1999 World Health Organization–International Society of Hypertension (WHO-ISH) committee, the 2003 European Society of Cardiology and Society of Hypertension committees, and in special situations or as possible alternative initial therapy, by the Sixth and Seventh Joint National Committees (JNC) on Prevention, Detection, Evaluation, and Treatment of High Blood Pressure. The JNC 7 suggests that the combination of an ACE inhibitor and a diuretic is appropriate initial therapy in some situations.

ACE Inhibitor Trials

During the past 3 to 4 years, several studies have helped to clarify the role of these agents in the management of hypertension.

■ HOPE

The Heart Outcomes Prevention Evaluation (HOPE) trial compared the results of treatment of a high-risk group of subjects ≥55 years of age who were being treated with multiple medications plus placebo to a group treated with an ACE inhibitor (ramipril 10 mg/day) plus other medications over 5 years. More than 9000 subjects were studied, 80% of whom had some evidence of cardiovascular (CV) disease or diabetes plus at least one other risk factor. While this was not specifically a study of hypertensive patients, 46% had hypertension. Differences in casual BP between the ACE inhibitor and the non–ACE inhibitor groups were –3/–2 mm Hg. In a small subset of 38 patients, ambulatory BPs in the ACE inhibitor group were considerably lower than in the control group. This was especially true of nocturnal BP.

At the end of the trial, 651 of 4645 patients in the ACE inhibitor group and 826 of the 4652 subjects in the non–ACE inhibitor group had died of CV disease, MI, or stroke (death rates were 8.1% in the control group and 6.1% in the ACE inhibitor group). MI and stroke rates were 12.3% compared with 9.9% and 4.9% compared with 3.4% in the placebo and ramipril groups, respectively. All reductions in CV events were significant between the groups. The BP differences were not believed to be great enough to account for all of the benefit. The ambulatory BP differences in a group of patients (who may have differed from a majority of the subjects in the HOPE study) may, however, be consistent with the decrease in CV events.

12

This trial suggests that in patients at very high risk for CV events, the addition of an ACE inhibitor (in this case, ramipril) to other medications reduces morbidity and mortality. Whether these results represent a class action or are specific to certain types of ACE inhibitors has not been settled. It is also possible that specific studies with other agents, such as the β-blockers or angiotensin II receptor blockers (ARBs) (which decrease the activity of the renin-angiotensin-aldosterone system [RAAS]), might produce similar results. Studies are ongoing to make this determination.

■ CAPPP

Results from the 5-year ACE inhibitor (Captopril Prevention Project [CAPPP]) study, which was a multicenter, randomized, prospective open trial in which investigators were unaware of the occurrence of end points, included more than 10,000 patients with hypertension and a supine diastolic blood pressure (DBP) >100 mm Hg. The study compared the ACE inhibitor captopril 50 to 100 mg daily (with hydrochlorothiazide and, in some cases, diltiazem added, if necessary) to a regimen of a β-blocker or a diuretic or a combination of both drugs (with diltiazem added, if necessary). There are no specific data regarding the exact number of subjects in the captopril group who required the addition of the thiazide or the number of subjects in the other treatment group who received both a β-blocker and a diuretic, but the percentage of subjects on combined therapy was high.

Results can be seen in **Figures 12.2** and **12.3**:

- All-cause mortality and relative risk of CV events were similar in both groups (difference not significant) (**Figure 12.2**).
- The occurrence of stroke appeared to be more common in the captopril-based treatment group
- Some differences in baseline characteristics (poor randomization) may explain some of these

FIGURE 12.2 — COMPARISON OF CAPTOPRIL-BASED AND β-BLOCKER/DIURETIC-BASED TREATMENT GROUPS IN THE MANAGEMENT OF HYPERTENSION (CAPPP STUDY)

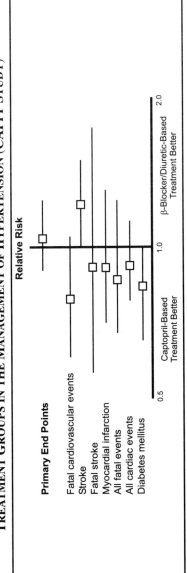

Abbreviation: CAPPP, Captopril Prevention Project [study].

No significant difference in overall cardiovascular events between angiotensin-converting enzyme (ACE) inhibitor (captopril)— and β-blocker–based treatment groups, except in the occurrence of diabetes (ACE inhibitor group better) or in the occurrence of stroke (β-blocker group better).

Adapted from: *Lancet.* 1999;353:611-615.

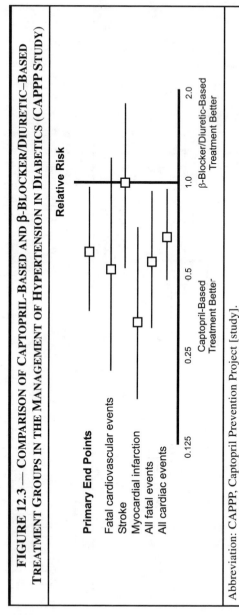

FIGURE 12.3 — COMPARISON OF CAPTOPRIL-BASED AND β-BLOCKER/DIURETIC-BASED TREATMENT GROUPS IN THE MANAGEMENT OF HYPERTENSION IN DIABETICS (CAPPP STUDY)

Abbreviation: CAPPP, Captopril Prevention Project [study].

Significant differences in outcome between angiotensin-converting enzyme (ACE) inhibitor (Captopril)– and β-blocker–based treatment groups in diabetic subjects.

Adapted from: *Lancet.* 1999;353:611-615.

findings, ie, initial BP was higher in the captopril group, which may explain the differences in stroke. There was, however, a higher percentage of patients with baseline evidence of ischemic heart disease in the β-blocker group. This may have favored the outcome vis-à-vis CV disease events with the ACE inhibitor.

- In the patients with diabetes, the occurrence of MI and all fatal and cardiac events were reduced to a greater extent in the captopril-based treatment group (**Figure 12.3**).

- Finally, *the incidence of new-onset diabetes was lower in the captopril group.*

Data from this trial as well as others suggest that an ACE inhibitor–based treatment program will reduce CV events (except possibly stroke) to as great a degree as a β-blocker/diuretic–based program and to a greater degree in diabetics. This finding is consistent with recent recommendations that an ACE inhibitor be part of a treatment program in most diabetic subjects.

■ UKPDS

In contrast to the CAPPP trial, an 8.4-year trial in Great Britain (United Kingdom Prospective Diabetes Study [UKPDS] 39) reported no difference in outcome between a captopril (ACE inhibitor)- and an atenolol (β-blocker)-based treatment program in type 2 non–insulin-dependent diabetics. The most important finding in the UKPDS reaffirmed the concept that tighter BP control compared with less-rigorous control (differences in BP between groups of –10/–5 mm Hg) makes a difference. Stroke, heart failure, and death related to diabetes were all reduced significantly in the group with better BP control.

In this study, patients who achieved BP levels of 144/82 mm Hg had a decrease of 44% in stroke, 56% in heart failure, and 32% in deaths related to diabetes when compared with those subjects with an achieved BP of 154/87 mm Hg (**Table 12.2**). Both microvascular (proteinuria, retinopathy) and macrovascular (stroke, coronary heart disease [CHD]) events were reduced by better BP control. As repeatedly noted, the results of the UKPDS should reduce the concern that some physicians may have had about using a β-blocker in subjects with diabetes. These also suggest that, at least in this study, it is the degree of BP lowering that makes most of the difference, not the medication used.

■ STOP-Hypertension-2

The Swedish Trial in Old Persons With Hypertension 2 (STOP-Hypertension-2) compared an ACE inhibitor– or calcium channel blocker (CCB)–based

---

TABLE 12.2 — COMPARATIVE STUDY OF ACE INHIBITOR– AND β-BLOCKER–BASED TREATMENT PROGRAM IN UKPDS

- Number of patients in study (non–insulin-dependent diabetics): 1148
- Tight blood pressure control; achieved blood pressure of 144/82 mm Hg compared with group with blood pressure of 154/87 mm Hg
- Reduction in cardiovascular risk—tight: less-effective blood pressure control
- Reduction in events:
  – Strokes 44%
  – Heart failure 56%
  – Deaths related to diabetes 32%
  – Microvascular disease 37%
  – Myocardial infarction and sudden death ..... 21% (not significant)
- No difference in outcome between different treatment groups; difference in achieved blood pressure accounted for difference in outcome.

Abbreviation: ACE, angiotensin-converting enzyme; UKPDS, United Kingdom Prospective Diabetes Study.

---

treatment program in 6614 people with an average age of 76 years with baseline BP of 194/98 mm Hg to a β-blocker/diuretic–treated group. At the end of 4 to 5 years, there was no difference in morbidity or mortality outcome between the "older" and "newer" drugs (**Figure 12.4**). BP was reduced to a similar degree in both groups to levels of 159/81 mm Hg. The overall results of this trial, as in the UKPDS, suggest that it is the degree of BP lowering that determines outcome and, in most cases, not the specific drug used.

The Blood Pressure Lowering Treatment Trialists collaboration performed separate meta-analyses of trials comparing ACE inhibitor– or CCB-based regimens with those based on a diuretic and/or β-blocker program and concluded that there were no differences in CV end points between the two groups.

While there was no significant difference in total, CV, and stroke mortality between the ACE inhibitor and CCB groups in the STOP-Hypertension-2 trial, the frequency of MI morbidity and mortality and CHF was less in the ACE inhibitor group compared with the CCB-treated patients (**Table 12.3** and **Figure 12.5**), suggesting that the ACE inhibitors were more effective in reducing MI and congestive heart failure (CHF) than the CCB-based treatment program. These findings are consistent with several smaller trials, ie, the Fosinopril Versus Amlodipine Cardiovascular Events Trial (FACET) and the Appropriate Blood Pressure Control in Diabetes (ABCD) study.

12

■ **Comparative Trials With ACE Inhibitors, Diuretics, and CCBs**
The Antihypertensive and Lipid-Lowering Treatment to Prevent Heart Attack Trial (ALLHAT)

ALLHAT is a landmark trial and represented the largest single study of hypertensive individuals ever undertaken. It was the first major long-term outcome trial directly comparing a diuretic-based treatment pro-

FIGURE 12.4 — SWEDISH TRIAL IN OLD PERSONS WITH HYPERTENSION 2 (STOP-HYPERTENSION-2): EFFECTS OF DRUG THERAPY ON MORTALITY AND MORBIDITY IN THE ELDERLY

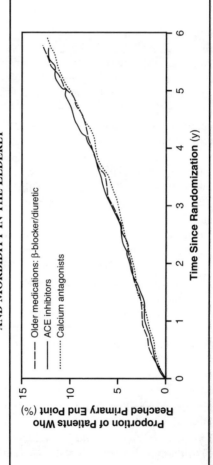

Hansson L, et al. *Lancet*. 1999;354:1751-1756.

TABLE 12.3 — STOP-HYPERTENSION-2 STUDY: FREQUENCY OF EVENTS PER 1000 PATIENT-YEARS			
	β-Blocker/Diuretic Group	ACE Inhibitor Group	Calcium Antagonist Group
Total mortality	33.1	34.4	32.8
Cardiovascular mortality	19.8	20.5	19.2
MI mortality and morbidity	14.1	12.8*	16.7*
Stroke mortality and morbidity	22.2	20.2	19.5
Frequency of diabetes mellitus	10.0	9.6	9.9
Frequency of CHF	16.4	13.9*	17.5*

Abbreviations: ACE, angiotensin-converting enzyme; CHF, congestive heart failure; MI, myocardial infarction; STOP, Swedish Trial in Old Patients With Hypertension.

* Significance between ACE and calcium channel blocker.

Hansson L, et al. *Lancet.* 1999;354:1751-1756.

12

FIGURE 12.5 — RELATIVE RISK OF CARDIOVASCULAR MORTALITY AND MORBIDITY WITH ACE INHIBITORS VS CALCIUM ANTAGONISTS IN STOP-HYPERTENSION-2 STUDY

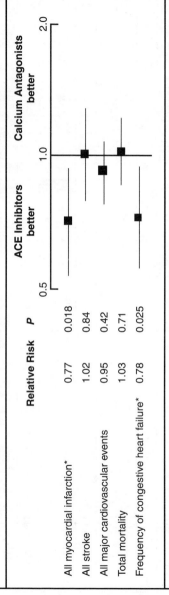

	Relative Risk	P
All myocardial infarction*	0.77	0.018
All stroke	1.02	0.84
All major cardiovascular events	0.95	0.42
Total mortality	1.03	0.71
Frequency of congestive heart failure*	0.78	0.025

Abbreviations: ACE, angiotensin-converting enzyme; STOP-Hypertension-2, Swedish Trial in Old Persons with Hypertension 2.

* Significant differences: ACE inhibitor group had fewer MI and CHF events than CCB group.

Hansson L, et al. *Lancet.* 1999;354:1751-1756.

gram with a CCB, an ACE inhibitor, and an α-blocker. More than 40,000 hypertensive patients with a mean age of 67 years with at least one other CHD risk factor were followed for >5 years. Thirty six percent of patients were diabetics (approximately 14,000); 35% were black. After all previous medications were stopped, patients were randomly assigned in a blinded fashion to treatment with a diuretic (chlorthalidone), a β-blocker, a CCB (amlodipine), an ACE inhibitor (lisinopril), and an α-blocker (doxazosin). Doses could be increased and additional drugs from other classes added in an effort to achieve goal BP. The additional drugs, however, were limited to nonstudy drugs, ie, if a patient had not reached goal BP on increasing doses of a diuretic, then a β-blocker, clonidine, methyldopa, reserpine, or hydralazine could be added. If patients failed to respond to the ACE inhibitor, a β-blocker or other drugs could be added, but a diuretic or a CCB could not. Thus there were some limitations to the approach of add-on therapy. The ALLHAT protocol, therefore, may not reflect what physicians do in their practices. However, about 24% of patients in both the CCB and ACE inhibitor groups did receive a diuretic during this study.

At the beginning of the study, <30% of hypertensive patients had been controlled at goal BP of ≤140/90 mm Hg; >90% of them were receiving some kind of antihypertensive therapy prior to entry into the study.

As noted, the α-blocker (doxazosin)/diuretic comparison arm of the trial was stopped after 3 years. Results had indicated that patients in this group had experienced 25% more CV events with a doubling of CHF compared with those in the thiazide-diuretic group.

After 5 years of follow-up, of the remaining 33,000 patients, >90% had attained goal DBP of <90 mm Hg and 67% had achieved systolic blood pressure (SBP) of <140 mm Hg. These results were achieved by following a fixed protocol that included a careful follow-up and demonstrated that hypertensive patients can achieve better control than suggested by national statistics in a practice setting if preestablished guidelines are utilized. Previous data suggested control of DBP in 60% to 70% of patients with a lesser degree of control of SBP. Careful attention to the achievement of goal BP, even with the use of possibly less than optimal add-on medication, will control BP at goal levels in a relatively high percentage of patients—an important message.

Data indicated that there were no differences in the primary outcome of fatal or nonfatal CHD events and no mortality difference between the ACE inhibitor, CCB, and diuretic groups (**Figure 12.6**). However, patients receiving the diuretic experienced fewer overall CV events than those on the other agents. Patients on diuretics had a lower incidence of heart failure and stroke than the group randomized to lisinopril (**Figures 12.7** and **12.8**). This was especially true in black patients where there were 40% fewer strokes in the diuretic-treated patients (most of the specific benefits attributed to diuretics were noted in the black subjects). The differences in risk of hospitalization and fatal heart failure were not, however, statistically significant (**Figure 12.9**). The diuretics were more effective in reducing the occurrence of hospitalization and fatal heart failure than amlodipine.

In ALLHAT, there was some difference in achieved BP among the three drugs tested. On average, SBP was 4 mm Hg less with diuretics than with lisinopril in black subjects and 3 mm Hg less in patients ≥65 years old. Overall, SBP was 2 mm Hg higher in the ACE inhibitor group compared with the diuretic cohort. These results were not unexpected, given the demographics of the patients studied, and could partially explain the differences in outcome. As noted, black subjects and the elderly generally experienced a greater decrease in BP on diuretics compared with

FIGURE 12.6 — NONFATAL MYOCARDIAL INFARCTION AND CORONARY HEART DISEASE DEATHS: SUBGROUP COMPARISONS (ALLHAT)

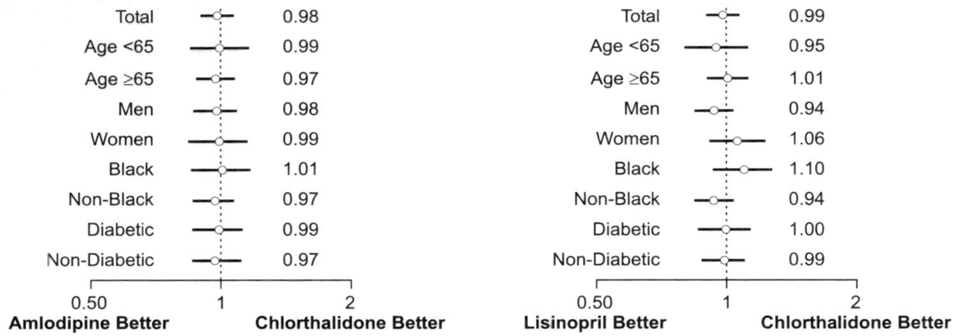

	Amlodipine Better — Chlorthalidone Better		Lisinopril Better — Chlorthalidone Better
Total	0.98	Total	0.99
Age <65	0.99	Age <65	0.95
Age ≥65	0.97	Age ≥65	1.01
Men	0.98	Men	0.94
Women	0.99	Women	1.06
Black	1.01	Black	1.10
Non-Black	0.97	Non-Black	0.94
Diabetic	0.99	Diabetic	1.00
Non-Diabetic	0.97	Non-Diabetic	0.99

Abbreviation: ALLHAT, Antihypertensive and Lipid-Lowering Treatment to Prevent Heart Attack Trial.

No statistically significant differences in the primary end points were noted with the three different medications tested.

The ALLHAT Officers and Coordinators for the ALLHAT Collaborative Research Group. *JAMA.* 2002:288:2981-2997.

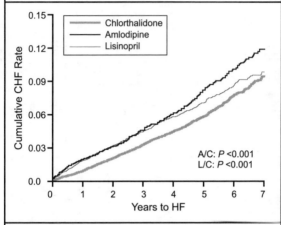

FIGURE 12.7 — CUMULATIVE EVENT RATES FOR HEART FAILURE BY ALLHAT TREATMENT GROUP

A/C: *P* <0.001
L/C: *P* <0.001

Abbreviations: A/C, amlodipine vs chlorthalidone; ALLHAT, Antihypertensive and Lipid-Lowering Treatment to Prevent Heart Attack Trial; CHF, congestive heart failure; HF, heart failure; L/C, lisinopril vs chlorthalidone.

Chlorthalidone was significantly more effective in reducing the occurrence of hospitalization and fatal heart failure than amlodipine.

The ALLHAT Officers and Coordinators for the ALLHAT Collaborative Research Group. *JAMA*. 2002;288:2981-2997.

medications that block the RAAS. The SBP was +0.8 mm Hg and the DBP –0.8 mm Hg with amlodipine compared with chlorthalidone. These results are similar to those noted in other comparative studies.

ALLHAT results have been criticized because of the protocol design. The ALLHAT protocol is not the usual one followed in practice and may have contributed, at least partially, to the difference in outcome. For example, if a diuretic had been routinely added to the ACE inhibitor, the difference in BP between groups probably would have been less; this combination usu-

FIGURE 12.8 — STROKE: SUBGROUP COMPARISONS (ALLHAT)

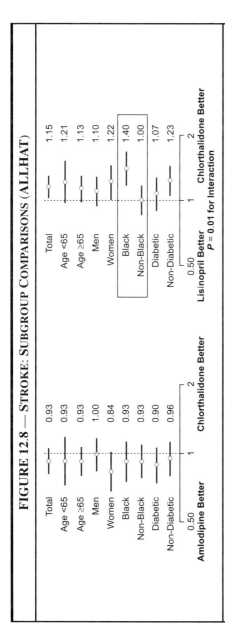

Abbreviation: ALLHAT, Antihypertensive and Lipid-Lowering Treatment to Prevent Heart Attack Trial.

For stroke, there was a significant differential effect by race, with $P = 0.01$. The relative risks (lisinopril vs chlorthalidone) for stroke were 1.40 ($P < 0.001$) in blacks and 1.00 ($P = 0.96$) in nonblacks.

The ALLHAT Officers and Coordinators for the ALLHAT Collaborative Research Group. *JAMA.* 2002;288:2981-2997.

FIGURE 12.9 — SIGNIFICANT CLINICAL OUTCOMES IN THE ALLHAT

	Amlodipine vs Chlorthalidone		Lisinopril vs Chlorthalidone	
	RR	P Value	RR	P Value
Primary Outcome				
CHD	0.98	NS	0.99	0.81
Secondary Outcomes				
Combined CVD		NS		NS
ESRD		NS		NS
All-cause mortality		NS		NS
Stroke		NS	1.15*	0.02*
Combined CVD	1.00	0.04	1.10	<0.001
Heart failure	1.36	<0.001	1.19	<0.001
Hospitalized/fatal heart failure	1.35	<0.001		NS
Angina (hospitalized or treated)		NS	1.11	0.01

Abbreviations: ALLHAT, Antihypertensive and Lipid-Lowering Treatment to Prevent Heart Attack Trial; CVD, cardiovascular disease; CHD, coronary heart disease; ESRD, end-stage renal disease; NS, no significant difference; RR, relative risk.

* Significant difference.

The ALLHAT Officers and Coordinators for the ALLHAT Collaborative Research Group. *JAMA.* 2002;288:2981-2997.

ally reduces or eliminates any difference in response to ACE inhibitors between black patients and white patients. It is also possible that any difference in outcome between the ACE inhibitor–based and diuretic-based treatment groups would have been minimized, especially the difference in heart failure events. In addition, patients on a CCB were not supposed to be given either a diuretic or an ACE inhibitor as a second agent. Again, it is possible that if a diuretic could have been given to more patients on the CCB, the differences in heart failure occurrence would have been minimized. Despite this lack of more logical choices of second-step medications, however, a large number of patients achieved goal BP.

The ALLHAT results appeared to have settled the debate about the benefits or risks of diuretics in the management of hypertension and played a role in the formulations of the JNC 7 guidelines, ie, recommendations for a thiazide diuretic to be used as initial therapy in most patients unless there was a compelling or specific reason to use another medication.

The ALLHAT results should not have been a major surprise since abundant data had previously demonstrated the effectiveness of diuretics in lowering BP and decreasing CV events even in the elderly and high-risk patients. New guidelines in JNC 7 indicate that these medications should not be limited to low-risk patients.

The Australian National Blood Pressure Trial

Another recent study, the Australian National Blood Pressure (ANBP 2) study, appeared to question the ALLHAT conclusions. This was a prospective, 4-year, randomized but *open-label* study with blinded assessment of end point in more than 6000 hypertensive subjects who were 65 to 84 years of age (mean age 72). Ninety-five percent of the patients were white. BP changes in an ACE inhibitor–based and a diuretic-based regimen were similar. At the end of the trial,

>20% of patients in both the ACE inhibitor and thiazide groups were on CCBs, 10% were on β-blockers, and 13% were on ARBs. This trial reported that an ACE inhibitor–based regimen was at least marginally more effective ($P = 0.05$) than a diuretic-based regimen in reducing morbidity and mortality outcome in hypertensive subjects (**Figure 12.10**).

But there were some problems with the ANBP 2 study. Importantly, it was *not blinded* and only 60% of patients remained on the initial study drug. More than 25% of patients crossed over from diuretics to the ACE inhibitor and vice versa. Although the ACE inhibitor–based group in this trial experienced fewer overall CV events than the diuretic group, the benefit occurred only in male patients ($P = 0.02$). There were no statistically significant differences in outcome between the ACE inhibitor and diuretics in women ($P = 0.98$). This is difficult to explain. The fact that there were few black patients in the ANBP 2 trial tended to favor the ACE inhibitor arm; in ALLHAT, the presence of one third black subjects tended to favor diuretics. Primary end points in ALLHAT only included CHD events. In ANBP 2, all CV events were included.

It is easy to criticize the ANBP 2 trial; fault can also be found with ALLHAT. A perfect trial has not been designed or carried out. But are the results of ALLHAT and ANBP 2 truly different? Can we believe the results of both studies with some qualifications? We believe so.

The ANBP 2 confirmed that an ACE inhibitor–based regimen essentially reduced CHD events and death to a marginally greater degree than a thiazide diuretic–based program. Numerous trials prior to ALLHAT had reported that ACE inhibitors and CCBs reduced morbidity and mortality in hypertensive patients with or without diabetes and/or renal disease. ALLHAT did not report that these agents should not

FIGURE 12.10 — RESULTS OF THE AUSTRALIAN NATIONAL BLOOD PRESSURE 2 TRIAL

End Point	Relative Risk ACE/Diuretic	P Value	ACE Inhibitors Superior ⟷ Diuretics Superior
All Subjects			0.2 — 1.0 — 5.0
All cardiovascular events or death from any cause	0.89	0.05	
First cardiovascular event or death from any cause	0.89	0.06	
Death from any cause	0.90	0.27	
Male Subjects			0.2 — 1.0 — 5.0
All cardiovascular events or death from any cause	0.83	0.02	
First cardiovascular event or death from any cause	0.83	0.02	
Death from any cause	0.83	0.14	
Female Subjects			0.2 — 1.0 — 5.0
All cardiovascular events or death from any cause	1.00	0.98	
First cardiovascular event or death from any cause	1.00	0.98	
Death from any cause	1.01	0.94	

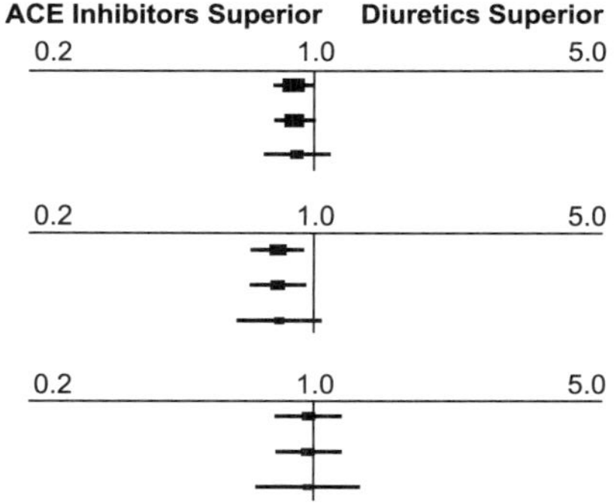

Abbreviation: ACE, angiotensin-converting enzyme.

Primary end points among all subjects, male subjects, and female subjects in comparative trial of an ACE inhibitor-based compared with a diuretic-based treatment regimen.

Wing LMH, et al. *N Engl J Med.* 2003;348:583-592.

be used, that they were dangerous, or that they were not effective.

The recent guidelines appear to reflect a reasonable approach to this debate. The JNC 7 utilized outcome evidence and not surrogate end points, not only from ALLHAT but from many other trials, in formulating its recommendations to continue diuretics as one of the cornerstones of treatment; it certainly did not ignore the other effective medications in their recommendations.

In deciding on specific therapies, the above data, as well as information from other trials regarding the use of ACE inhibitors, should be considered.

The PROGRESS Trial

Results from the Perindopril Protection Against Recurrent Stroke Study (PROGRESS), a double-blind trial in more than 6000 patients who had suffered a stroke or transient ischemic attack (TIA), have helped answer an important question. Data regarding the use of antihypertensive medications in this type of patient had not definitely established benefit of treatment. In PROGRESS, the use of an ACE inhibitor (perindopril) with a diuretic (indapamide) resulted in a decrease in BP of 12/5 mm Hg and a significant reduction of 43% in recurrent strokes (both ischemic and hemorrhagic) when compared with standard therapy. The combination ACE inhibitor/diuretic was effective whereas the ACE inhibitor alone was not (**Figure 12.11**). This important observation suggests that patients with evidence of cerebrovascular disease and even minimal elevation of BP should be treated with an ACE inhibitor/diuretic combination. It is possible that the same results could be obtained with an ARB/diuretic combination, but currently, there are no specific data available for confirmation. The use of a combination RAAS-blocking agent and a diuretic appears to be an

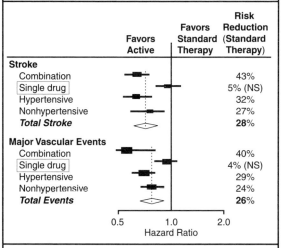

FIGURE 12.11 — EFFECTS OF AN ACE INHIBITOR (PERINDOPRIL) AND A DIURETIC (INDAPAMIDE) ON STROKES AND VASCULAR EVENTS

	Favors Active	Favors Standard Therapy	Risk Reduction (Standard Therapy)
Stroke			
Combination			43%
Single drug			5% (NS)
Hypertensive			32%
Nonhypertensive			27%
Total Stroke			**28%**
Major Vascular Events			
Combination			40%
Single drug			4% (NS)
Hypertensive			29%
Nonhypertensive			24%
Total Events			**26%**

0.5   1.0   2.0
Hazard Ratio

Abbreviations: ACE, angiotensin-converting enzyme; NS, not significant.

Patients on a single medication did not experience a decrease in either stroke or cardiovascular events. Patients on combination perindopril/indapamide noted a significant benefit.

Modified from: PROGRESS Collaborative Group. *Lancet.* 2001;358:1033-1041.

effective approach to management of a patient with a previous cerebrovascular accident.

Summary

It should be remembered that goal BP is not achieved in many patients with an ACE inhibitor or an ARB without the concurrent use of a diuretic.

If an ACE inhibitor is used as first-step monotherapy in certain patients, small doses should be prescribed initially (**Table 12**.1); the maximum suggested doses in this table may be lower than those recommended in the manufacturer's prescribing information. Rather than increasing dosage to a maximum, we prefer to add a small dose of a diuretic if target BP is not achieved with a minimal or, at most, moderate dose of an ACE inhibitor. This is similar to our approach to therapy with other medications. For example, if a patient is taking enalapril or lisinopril 10 mg/day or captopril 50 mg/bid and BP has not normalized, a diuretic should probably be added. Here is another instance where combination therapy with one of the many available medications should be considered. There are several available combinations of an ACE inhibitor and a diuretic (**Table 5**.6).

Side Effects

Side effects of the ACE inhibitors are relatively uncommon, except for cough. Most patients tolerate these agents well and quality of life is not compromised; in fact, some people clearly feel better on these medications. Several adverse reactions have been noted:

- About 15% to 20% of patients develop a dry, hacking cough that is persistent and annoying. If it is recognized early, patients can be saved the trouble of going through extensive diagnostic evaluations for various types of allergies, bronchitis, or pulmonary disease. The cough will usually, but not always, disappear in 3 to 5 days on cessation of the medication. It is reported to be more common in women, but in our experience, almost an equal number of men and women develop it. The etiology is unknown, but it may be related to increased levels of bradykinin or substance P. The fact that cough is rare in patients receiving an ARB that has no effect on the bradykinin system is suggestive evidence that excess bradykinin is related to this adverse effect.

- Postural hypotension and dizziness may occur, especially in patients already receiving a diuretic and in the elderly.
- Angioedema is rare but can be serious; there is an acute onset of difficulty in breathing or swallowing with swelling of the lips, etc. It usually occurs within several days to 1 week of institution of therapy and most often clears quickly when therapy is discontinued.
- A macular rash is occasionally seen (in <2% to 3% of cases).
- Loss of taste and appetite is uncommon but does occur, especially in older people (it is rare with ACE inhibitors other than captopril). Symptoms may be subtle and weight loss can result if medicine is not discontinued within a short time. It may take >2 weeks for taste to return to normal.

ACE inhibitors or ARBs should not be given to pregnant women, and these medications should be discontinued if a patient becomes pregnant. Medications that interfere with the RAAS may cause fetal and neonatal morbidity and death when administered to pregnant women.

Although the manufacturer's prescribing information suggests that diuretics be stopped prior to the addition of an ACE inhibitor, a different strategy is effective and safe: the diuretic dosage can be reduced by about one half and the ACE inhibitor started in small doses. In some cases, measures of renal function (ie, blood urea nitrogen [BUN] or creatinine levels) rise following the institution of therapy with an ACE inhibitor, especially if a diuretic is being used concurrently. This occurs not only in patients with bilateral renal artery stenosis but also in others, especially older people who undoubtedly have some nephrosclerotic changes.

ACE Inhibitors and Renovascular Disease

The reason for the possible deterioration of renal function in patients with bilateral narrowing of the renal arteries and renovascular hypertension when they are given an ACE inhibitor is that in these patients, BP often is dependent on high levels of angiotensin II. A decrease in renal blood flow from the arterial stenosis increases renin release, which leads to an increase in angiotensin II in an attempt to maintain an adequate pressure and flow in the renal arteries. ACE inhibition reduces angiotensin II levels, decreases BP and intrarenal pressure, and may significantly reduce renal blood flow and lead to an increase in creatinine levels. Simple measures of renal function (ie, BUN and creatinine levels) should be checked within 1 to 2 months after beginning ACE inhibitor therapy; if a *marked* change occurs, therapy should be reevaluated.

Although it was originally believed that ACE inhibitors would only be effective in hypertensive patients with high renin levels, this has not proved to be true. Although these medications are more effective in patients with high-renin hypertension (about 15% to 20% of all hypertensives), they will also lower BP in many patients with normal or low renin levels. As noted elsewhere (see Chapter 2, *Diagnosis*), measurement of renin levels has not been recommended as an initial diagnostic procedure. We find it of little value in choosing an appropriate mode of therapy.

ACE inhibitors have been found to be especially effective as antihypertensive agents in young and middle-aged whites. They are less effective in blacks and, in some instances, may be less effective in the elderly. Normal BP levels will be achieved in about

30% to 40% of patients with stage 1 or stage 2 uncomplicated hypertension when an ACE inhibitor is used as monotherapy. However, as repeatedly emphasized, when a small dose of a diuretic is added to an ACE inhibitor, a goal BP of <140/90 mm Hg will be achieved in approximately 75% to 80% of patients, regardless of race or age.

Some data have demonstrated that ACE inhibitors may decrease insulin resistance. This effect provides a possible theoretical reason to use these agents in preferential subsets of hypertensive patients (eg, those who are obese or have elevated triglyceride levels and low high-density lipoprotein [HDL] levels) (metabolic syndrome). These patients probably have increased insulin resistance and are at risk for type 2 diabetes. Data from the CAPPP study suggest that this may be appropriate therapy in at least some of these subjects. Data from the HOPE study also suggest that in very high-risk subjects, an ACE inhibitor should be part of the regimen to prevent further CV events. More data are necessary before a definitive recommendation can be made. The use of an ACE inhibitor (most often with a diuretic and/or a β-blocker) will slow progression of renal failure in subjects with type 1 diabetic neuropathy. These agents should be considered drugs of choice in these patients.

Comparative Data With ACE Inhibitors and Calcium Channel Blockers

Several recent randomized prospective studies have compared the effects of an ACE inhibitor with those of a long-acting CCB in patients with type 2 (non–insulin-dependent) diabetes. The 3.5-year Fosinopril Versus Amlodipine Cardiovascular Events Trial (FACET), a comparative study of an ACE inhibitor (fosinopril) and a CCB (amlodipine) reported that BP changes were greater with amlodipine (–18/–8 mm

Hg) than with fosinopril (–13/–8 mm Hg), but there were no differences between the drugs in changes in lipids, plasma insulin, or HbA_{IC} levels. Numbers of events were small, but major vascular events were significantly different between fosinopril and amlodipine, 14/189 patients compared with 27/191 patients, respectively. While there were trends in reduction of specific vascular events, such as fatal and nonfatal MI or hospitalization for angina in the ACE group compared with the CCB group, these did not achieve statistical significance (**Table 12.4**). However, as noted, the difference between the two treatments in the occurrence of all major CV events was significant.

The Appropriate Blood Pressure Control in Diabetes (ABCD) study was a 5-year randomized blinded trial in non–insulin-dependent diabetics. A long-acting CCB (nisoldipine) was given to 235 patients, and 235 patients received an ACE inhibitor (enalapril). Both drugs showed similar control of BP, with no significant differences in blood glucose and lipid levels, but

TABLE 12.4 — CARDIOVASCULAR EVENTS IN THE FACET STUDY*		
Event	Fosinopril (189 patients)	Amlodipine (191 patients)
Fatal/nonfatal stroke	4	5
Fatal/nonfatal MI	10	13
Hospitalized for angina	0	4
Any major CV event	14[†]	27[†]
Abbreviations: CV, cardiovascular; FACET, Fosinopril Versus Amlodipine Cardiovascular Events Trial; MI, myocardial infarction.		
* Mean age of patients 63 years; 3.5-year follow-up. † $P = 0.03$.		
From: *Diabetes Care*. 1998;21:597-603.		

the nisoldipine group experienced a statistically significant greater number of fatal and nonfatal MIs than the enalapril group (**Table 12.5**). Again, the numbers of events were small.

Thus both the FACET and the ABCD studies suggest that an ACE inhibitor–based regimen will reduce CV events to a greater degree than dihydropyridine-based treatment programs in non–insulin-dependent diabetics. However, neither of these studies provided evidence of harm from the CCB since events in *nontreated* type 2 diabetics appear to be similar to

TABLE 12.5 — ADJUSTED CARDIOVASCULAR EVENTS IN THE ABCD STUDY[*][†]		
Event	**Nisoldipine (235 patients)**	**Enalapril (235 patients)**
Fatal/nonfatal MI	25[‡]	5[‡]
Nonfatal MI	22[‡]	5[‡]
Cerebrovascular accidents	11	7
Congestive heart failure	6	5
Death from CV event	10	5
Death from any cause	17	13

Abbreviations: ABCD, Appropriate Blood Pressure Control in Diabetes; CV, cardiovascular; MI, myocardial infarction.

[*] 93 patients assigned to nisoldipine also needed a diuretic and 89 patients required a β-blocker to achieve goal blood pressure; in the enalapril group, 99 patients required a β-blocker and 110 patients required a diuretic to achieve goal blood pressure.
[†] 5-year follow-up.
[‡] Significant difference between groups.

Adapted from: *N Engl J Med*. 1998;338:645-652.

12

those treated with a CCB in the ABCD study; rather, these data suggest benefits for the use of an ACE inhibitor and reinforce the recommendations of the JNC 7 that an ACE inhibitor is indicated as part of a treatment program in the management of diabetic hypertensive individuals. In patients with hypertension and nondiabetic renal disease, an ACE inhibitor or another agent that blocks the RAAS (usually with a diuretic) may offer some advantages over other therapy in slowing down progression of renal disease. Some investigators still believe, however, that even in these patients, the degree of BP lowering and not specific therapy makes the difference. As noted, the STOP-Hypertension-2 study also suggested that an ACE inhibitor–based treatment program reduced CV events to a greater degree than a CCB-based program. The African American Study of Kidney Disease (AASK) results provide additional evidence that the use of an ACE inhibitor is more effective in preventing renal disease progression in black patients than a dihydropyridine CCB.

The ACE inhibitors represent a major advance in the management of hypertension. Their availability has led to an increased rate of control and has simplified management of many patients. We have used the ACE inhibitors most often in combination with a diuretic. To reemphasize, data suggest that ACE inhibitors should be part of the regimen in the treatment of diabetic hypertensive subjects and high-risk patients with CHD. They are suitable as initial therapy, usually with a small dose of a diuretic. The WHO-ISH and European reports on the management of hypertension also suggest that ACE inhibitors are appropriate as initial monotherapy (see Chapter 4, *Drug Treatment of Hypertension: General Information* and **Table 4.5**).

13 Angiotensin II Receptor Blockers

The angiotensin II receptor blockers (ARBs) have now been in use as antihypertensive agents for >5 years. These agents block the renin-angiotensin cascade more peripherally than the angiotensin-converting enzyme (ACE) inhibitors do and they do not interfere with the generation of angiotensin II. They block the action of this pressor substance at the receptor site, ie, blood vessel walls (**Figure 12**.**1**).

Seven ARBs have been approved by the Food and Drug Administration (FDA) for the treatment of hypertension (**Table 13**.**1**):

- Losartan (Cozaar)
- Valsartan (Diovan)
- Irbesartan (Avapro)
- Candesartan (Atacand)
- Eprosartan (Teveten)
- Telmisartan (Micardis)
- Olmesartan (Benicar).

13

Most studies indicate that these medications are as effective in lowering blood pressure (BP) as the ACE inhibitors when used as monotherapy.

The use of an ARB reduces vascular resistance without reducing cardiac output. Heart rate may be increased in some patients. No significant change in lipid and serum glucose levels is noted. Renal blood flow is maintained. This class of medication is well tolerated with few side effects; BP is lowered without the problem of cough that may occur when an ACE inhibitor is given. The ARBs do not interfere with the breakdown of bradykinin, ie, bradykinin levels are not increased.

TABLE 13.1—ANGIOTENSIN II RECEPTOR BLOCKERS USED FOR TREATING HYPERTENSION

Generic (Trade) Name	Usual Dosage Range		Adverse Reactions	Physiologic Effects	Comments
	Dose (mg)	Frequency			
Candesartan (Atacand)	8-32	1/day	Occasional dizziness; generally well tolerated	Blocks action of angiotensin II; → vasodilation; ↓ aldosterone secretion	Diuretic doses should be reduced before starting angiotensin II receptor blocker whenever possible to prevent excessive hypotension. Reduce dose in patients with serum creatinine >3.0 mg/dL. Can cause renal failure in patients with bilateral renal artery stenosis
Eprosartan (Teveten)	400-800	1 or 2/day			
Irbesartan (Avapro)	150-300	1/day			
Losartan (Cozaar)	25-100	1 or 2/day			
Olmesartan (Benicar)	20-40	1/day			
Telmisartan (Micardis)	20-80	1/day			
Valsartan (Diovan)	80-320	1/day			

ARBs may interfere with other pathways since angiotensin II is not generated solely by the renin-angiotensin system. The exact significance of this effect is unknown at this time.

An increase in serum potassium is infrequent when these agents are used, possibly because aldosterone levels are not always decreased.

Data in patients with primary or essential hypertension suggest that the ARBs can increase the production and availability of nitric oxide (NO), a strong vasodilator substance, and decrease the vasoconstriction activity of endothelin on blood vessel walls. This may be an important effect since endothelial cell dysfunction (impaired vasodilation secondary to reduced NO) has been shown to be present in hypertensive individuals. *As with the ACE inhibitors, ARBs should not be administered to pregnant women.*

A review of published studies of ARBs in hypertensive patients indicates that there may be some added effect when the doses of these agents are increased from the starting dose (ie, dose-response curves may not be flat). A meta-analysis reported little difference in the efficacy of the different ARBs, but some data suggest that there is about a –3-5/–2-3 mm Hg difference in responses to increased dosages of many of these agents. A study with candesartan, for example, reported an overall further decrease of about 4-8/2-4 mm Hg when the dosage was increased from 16 to 32 mg/day. There may be some instances, therefore, when titration to a higher dose may be beneficial, such as from 50 to 100 mg of losartan, 150 to 300 mg of irbesartan, 16 to 32 mg of candesartan, 80 to 160 mg of valsartan, 40 to 80 mg of telmisartan, or 20 to 40 mg of olmesartan. Importantly, side effects are not usually increased with an increase in dosage.

Several recent trials (Reduction in End Points in Non–Insulin-Dependent Diabetes Mellitus With the Angiotensin II Antagonist Losartan [RENAAL] and Program for Irbesartan Morbidity and Mortality Evaluation [PRIME]) suggest that high doses (ie, 100 mg and 300 mg of the agents losartan and irbesartan, respectively) may be more effective than smaller doses in delaying progression of diabetic nephropathy (see *Angiotensin II Receptor Blockers in Special Situations* in this chapter). In most cases, however, best results will probably be obtained by limiting the use of these medications to the initial dosage and adding a small dose of a diuretic as a second step in the nonresponders or partial responders. In the recent trials, as in most other clinical trials, other medications were usually given with the study drug; in this instance, an ARB. Goal BP (a diastolic blood pressure [DBP] <90 mm Hg or a decrease of >10 mm Hg) is achieved in about 50% to 60% of patients when an ARB is used as monotherapy in initial, as well as in titrated, doses.

It is important to reemphasize that the BP-lowering effects of the ARBs, as with the ACE inhibitors, are greatly increased when a diuretic is added. Fixed-dose combinations are available and are effective in lowering BP in both young and elderly patients; combinations include:

- Losartan (50 mg or 100 mg) with hydrochlorothiazide (12.5 mg or 25 mg) (Hyzaar)
- Valsartan (80 mg or 160 mg) with hydrochlorothiazide (12.5 mg) (Diovan HCT)
- Irbesartan (150 mg or 300 mg) with hydrochlorothiazide (12.5 mg) (Avalide)
- Candesartan (16 mg or 32 mg) with hydrochlorothiazide (12.5 mg) (Atacand HCT)
- Telmisartan (40 mg or 80 mg) with hydrochlorothiazide (12.5 mg) (Micardis HCT)
- Eprosartan (600 mg) with hydrochlorothiazide (12.5 mg or 25 mg) (Teveten HCT)
- Olmesartan (20 mg or 40 mg) with hydrochlorothiazide (12.5 mg or 25 mg) (Benicar HCT).

These are also listed in **Table 15.6**. In black patients, ARBs as monotherapy are less effective than diuretics and calcium channel blockers (CCBs). However, as with the ACE inhibitors, when ARBs are combined with small doses of a diuretic, any racial differences in BP lowering or response rates are eliminated. This may be the most efficient way to use these agents, ie, begin combination therapy rather than titrating the dose upward if an initial dose does not result in goal BP. This may be particularly true in diabetic patients, since a majority of these patients, especially those with any evidence of renal disease, require more than one medication to achieve goal BP. Combination therapy may then be increased if necessary before adding another medication. More than 70% to 75% of patients will achieve goal BP when a low-dose combination of an ARB and a diuretic is used as initial therapy. The additional decrease in BP with combination therapy compared with initial starting-dose therapy with this new class of medication is approximately –6-8/–3-4 mm Hg.

As suggested in the Seventh Joint National Committee (JNC 7) on Prevention, Detection, Evaluation, and Treatment of High Blood Pressure report, this type of combination may be appropriate initial therapy in many hypertensive patients (ie, stage 2 hypertension or stage 1 hypertension with diabetes, etc). In the opinion of many investigators, the use of an ARB can be considered in the same situations that an ACE inhibitor is indicated: either as monotherapy in some situations or as part of a treatment program that includes a diuretic or other medications. This is based on the facts that ARBs:

- Are as effective antihypertensive agents as the ACE inhibitors
- Are well tolerated
- Reduce left ventricular hypertrophy (LVH) and proteinuria

- Have favorable hemodynamic effects in patients with heart failure
- Several of them have been shown to slow progression of renal disease in patients with type 2 diabetes and varying degrees of nephropathy (see specific studies below).

The use of an ARB or an ARB/diuretic combination may be preferred in some elderly patients who do not reach goal BP levels with a diuretic. These agents are well tolerated and will decrease systolic BP to a greater degree than DBP.

As noted, the World Health Organization–International Society of Hypertension (WHO-ISH) and the European Society committees have listed ARBs as possible initial therapy. This committee also states that effectiveness of this group of compounds, as well as other antihypertensive agents, is increased when given in combination with another agent with a different mechanism of action. While specific long-term outcome data regarding the reduction of cardiovascular (CV) events with ARBs are not as definitive as with some of the other classes of medications (except in diabetic patients with varying degrees of proteinuria and renal insufficiency), these recommendations seem reasonable.

Angiotensin II Receptor Blockers in Special Situations

Losartan has been shown to have favorable hemodynamic effects in patients with congestive heart failure (CHF). Valsartan has also been shown to have favorable hemodynamic effects in patients with CHF-reducing capillary wedge pressure, systemic vascular resistance, and plasma aldosterone levels. A long-term morbidity and mortality trial (Valsartan Heart Failure Trial [Val-HeFT]) has been completed. Results indicated that combined all-cause mortality and morbidity were reduced by 13% when valsartan was added to usual therapy, which included diuretics, ACE inhibitors, and, in most cases, digitalis. Hospital admissions for heart failure were decreased by 28%.

Additional findings from Val-HeFT suggest that morbidity outcome may be improved if valsartan is used along with an ACE inhibitor but may be worsened if it is added to a regimen that already includes an ACE inhibitor and a β-blocker. Since about 20% to 25% of patients with CHF are being treated with a β-blocker, this finding must be considered in management decisions. In the Candesartan in Heart Failure—Assessment of Reduction in Mortality and Morbidity (CHARM) trial, the use of candesartan, when added to a regimen that included an ACE inhibitor or as a substitute for an ACE inhibitor in patients with a decreased ejection fraction, reduced CV events and episodes of severe heart failure. Benefit was noted in patients receiving a β-blocker in addition to an ACE inhibitor as well as in those who were not. In subjects with a normal ejection fraction, benefit was not seen when the ARB was added to other therapy.

The Evaluation of Losartan in the Elderly-Part 2 [ELITE 2]) trial reported only minor differences in outcome between the addition of this agent or an ACE inhibitor when these agents were added to background therapy in the management of CHF. While this trial was interpreted as being negative, it suggests that an ARB can probably be used instead of an ACE inhibitor if the latter is not well tolerated in the management of CHF. The CHARM study results appear to confirm this finding.

The recently completed Losartan Intervention for Endpoint Reduction in Hypertension (LIFE) study reported that an ARB-based regimen (in a majority of patients, a diuretic was necessary to achieve goal BPs) was significantly more effective than a β-blocker–

13

based regimen in reducing stroke and new onset diabetes in patients with LVH. The incidence of myocardial infarctions (MIs) and CV mortality was not significantly different between drugs. In the hypertensive diabetic patient with LVH, however, a significant decrease in heart failure, all-cause mortality, and death from CV disease was noted in the patients treated with losartan compared with those in the atenolol treatment group (**Table 13**.**2**). The LIFE study, as well as other trials in hypertensive individuals, has demonstrated that the use of an ARB results in a greater degree of LVH regression than the use of a β-blocker.

What Role Do the ARBs Have in the Management of Diabetic Patients?

Increasing data suggest that the use of ARBs (in addition to other medications) produces beneficial effects in diabetic patients with microproteinuria. Several recent trials have compared the effects of an ARB with those of an ACE inhibitor, either alone or in combination, on BP and albuminuria in hypertensive diabetic subjects with microalbuminuria. One study (Candesartan and Lisinopril Microalbuminuria [CALM]) compared the ARB candesartan (16 mg qd) and the ACE inhibitor lisinopril (20 mg qd) as monotherapy or in combination in type 2 diabetics and reported that BP reduction and decrease in microproteinuria were similar with both drugs. The combination lowered BP further than monotherapy but did not improve proteinuria to a greater degree than each medication alone. Another trial reported similar reductions in microproteinuria with losartan and the ACE inhibitor enalapril. Studies in specific patient populations with ARBs alone and in combination with other medications, including ACE inhibitors, have also been reported.

TABLE 13.2 — LIFE STUDY IN DIABETES: RESULTS OF AN ARB-BASED (LOSARTAN) COMPARED WITH A β-BLOCKER–BASED (ATENOLOL) TREATMENT PROGRAM IN 1195 DIABETIC HYPERTENSIVE PATIENTS WITH LEFT VENTRICULAR HYPERTROPHY*

Event	Difference ARB/BB (%)
Achieved blood pressure (mm Hg)	-2/0[†]
Primary end point (CV mortality stroke, myocardial infarction)	-24[‡]
Death from CV disease	-37[‡]
Heart failure	-41[‡]
All-cause mortality	-39[‡]

Abbreviations: ARB, angiotensin II receptor blocker; BB, β blocker; CV, cardiovascular; LIFE, Losartan Intervention for Endpoint Reduction in Hypertension.

* No significant differences between medications in stroke and myocardial infarction.
† ARB, 146/79 mm Hg; BB, 148/79 mm Hg.
‡ Significant difference.

Lindholm LH et al. *Lancet.* 2002;359:1004-1010.

13

An important finding in comparative studies with ARBs as well as with ACE inhibitors is outlined in **Table 13.3**. In many major studies, the occurrence of new-onset diabetes has been less when a treatment regimen included an ARB or an ACE inhibitor compared with treatment with other agents. In these prospective studies, data differ somewhat from previous studies that indicated no difference in new-onset diabetes with various medications (see Chapter 5, *Diuretics*). As noted in the 5-year ALLHAT, the finding of more diabetes with chlorthalidone therapy, however, did not affect CV-event outcome.

TABLE 13.3 — EFFECT OF ANTIHYPERTENSIVE THERAPY ON NEW-ONSET DIABETES

Study	No. of Subjects	Ages	BP (mm/Hg)	TOD	Comment
LIFE	9193	55 to 85	174/98	LVH	Atenolol (β-blocker)–based therapy and losartan (ARB)–based therapy; HCTZ added; 25% lower incidence with losartan compared with atenolol
HOPE	5720	55+	139/99	High risk	ACE inhibitor (ramipril)–based therapy; other medications; 24% lower incidence in ACE inhibitor group
SCOPE	4964	70–89 (76*)	166/90	High risk	Candesartan (ARB)-based therapy; other medications; 20% trend to reduction of new-onset diabetes with candesartan
ALLHAT	33,000	67*	146/84	High risk	3.5% fewer cases of diabetes with lisinopril than with a diuretic-based treatment program
INVEST	>16,000	??	??	High risk	6.1% developed diabetes in CCB/ACE inhibitor–based treatment group compared with 7.2% in β-blocker/diuretic–based treatment group

Abbreviations: ACE, angiotensin-converting enzyme; ALLHAT, Antihypertensive and Lipid-Lowering Treatment to Prevent Heart Attack Trial; ARB, angiotensin II receptor blocker; BP, blood pressure; CCB, calcium channel blocker; HCTZ, hydrochlorothiazide; HOPE, Heart Outcomes Prevention Evaluation; INVEST, International Verapamil SR/Trandolapril Study; LIFE, Losartan Intervention for End-point Reduction in Hypertension; LVH, left ventricular hypertrophy; SCOPE, Study on Cognition and Prognosis in the Elderly; TOD, target-organ damage.

* Mean age.

13

■ RENAAL, IDNT, and IRMA 2 Studies

The results of three trials, RENAAL, Irbesartan Diabetic Nephropathy Trial (IDNT), and Irbesartan Microalbuminuria Type 2 Diabetes Mellitus in Hypertension Patients (IRMA 2) trial have been published. Both of the latter trials were part of the PRIME research program.

RENAAL

RENAAL was a 3-year multinational controlled trial evaluating the effects on renal function of an angiotensin II receptor antagonist, losartan (Cozaar) (50-100 mg/qd), when added to other medications in 1513 type 2 diabetic patients. Those on losartan were compared with similar patients whose therapy included antihypertensive medications other than an ACE inhibitor or an ARB (the "placebo" group). Patients had average baseline BP of 153/82 mm Hg with evidence of diabetic nephropathy with proteinuria (>500 mg/d) and mean baseline creatinine levels of 1.9 mg/dL. At the end of the trial, there was a significant reduction in the risk of renal disease progression, with fewer patients requiring renal dialysis or transplantation in the ARB group compared with the non–ARB-treated group. No difference in mortality or the total number of CV events was noted, but 32% ($P = 0.005$) fewer episodes of hospitalization for CHF were noted in the group receiving the ARB compared with patients who were treated with other agents.

This is the first study to specifically demonstrate a statistically significant decrease in progression to end-stage renal disease (ESRD) in patients with type 2 diabetic nephropathy. A 16% reduction in the composite end point—doubling of serum creatinine in ESRD and death—was noted. A 28% ($P = 0.002$) decrease in the occurrence of ESRD was noted in the group of patients treated with losartan (**Figure 13.1**). Studies with ACE inhibitor–based therapy had previ-

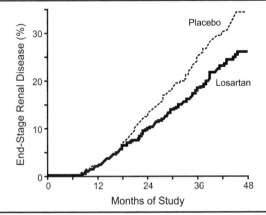

FIGURE 13.1 — KAPLAN-MEIER CURVES OF THE PERCENTAGE OF TYPE 2 DIABETIC PATIENTS WITH END-STAGE RENAL DISEASE IN THE RENAAL STUDY

Abbreviations: ACE, angiotensin-converting enzyme; ARB, angiotensin II receptor blocker; RENAAL, Reduction in Endpoints in Patients With Non–Insulin-Dependent Diabetes Mellitus With the Angiotensin II Antagonist Losartan [study].

Losartan graph line indicates therapy with ARB or other medications, while the placebo line shows therapy with medications other than an ARB or an ACE inhibitor. (Risk reduction, 28%; $P = 0.002$.)

Brenner BM, et al. *N Engl J Med.* 2001;345:865.

ously reported a reduction in progression of proteinuria in these patients but not a significant reduction in ESRD.

IDNT

IDNT compared results of treatment of three groups of subjects with type 2 diabetes, significant proteinuria, and evidence of renal function impairment.

One thousand seven hundred fifteen patients were randomized to receive 1) an ARB, irbesartan (Avapro) up to 300 mg/qd, in addition to medications other than an ACE inhibitor or a CCB; 2) amlodipine 2.5-10 mg/qd in addition to other medications other than the study drugs; or 3) a so-called placebo group who were taking medications other than the study drugs.

Mean duration of the study was 2.6 years. Primary end point of the study was a composite end point of development of ESRD, death from any cause, and the time to doubling of the serum creatinine concentration (**Figure 13**.2). Treatment with irbesartan plus other

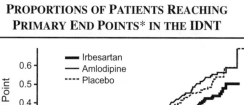

FIGURE 13.2 — CUMULATIVE PROPORTIONS OF PATIENTS REACHING PRIMARY END POINTS* IN THE IDNT

Abbreviation: IDNT, Irbesartan in Diabetic Nephropathy Trial.

Proportion of patients with primary end points. Differences between irbesartan and placebo and irbesartan and amlodipine were significant (–20% [$P = 0.02$] and –23% [$P = 0.006$], respectively).

* Doubling of baseline serum creatinine, end-stage renal disease, and death from any cause.

Lewis EJ, et al. *N Engl J Med*. 2001;345:856.

medications that did not include an ACE inhibitor, another ARB, or a CCB resulted in a significant 20% reduction in risk of the primary end point and 33% in the risk of doubling of serum creatinine compared with patients treated with medications other than an ARB, ACE inhibitor, or CCB ("placebo" group). Of importance was that a 23% reduction ($P = 0.006$) in the primary end point and a 37% reduction ($P = 0.001$) in the risk of doubling of creatinine was noted in the irbesartan group compared with subjects on amlodipine (plus other medications except ARBs, ACE inhibitors, or CCBs). Achieved BP differences between the ARB and CCB groups were not significant. Proteinuria was also significantly reduced in the irbesartan group compared with other therapies. No difference in all-cause mortality was noted among groups in this trial.

IRMA 2

The IRMA 2 trial compared the effects on patients of irbesartan (150 or 300 mg/day) plus other medications (other than ACE inhibitors or ARBs) with the effects on patients of medications other than an ARB or ACE inhibitor. Five hundred ninety type 2 diabetic patients who demonstrated microproteinuria (30-300 mg/day) were followed for 2 years. No significant differences in achieved BP were noted in the three groups of patients. There was a 70% reduction in progression to more severe renal disease in the group of patients treated with irbesartan; higher doses (300 mg) proved to be more effective than the 150-mg dose. The group that received irbesartan 300 mg/day compared with the non-ARB group experienced a significant reduction in the number of patients who progressed to frank proteinuria (>300 mg/day). In addition, in 34% of patients, the amount of albumin excreted normalized (**Figure 13.3**).

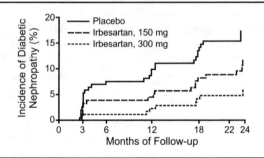

FIGURE 13.3 — PROGRESSION OF DIABETIC NEPHROPATHY IN IRMA 2 STUDY OF HYPERTENSIVE PATIENTS WITH TYPE 2 DIABETES AND MICROPROTEINURIA

Abbreviations: ACE, angiotensin-converting enzyme; ARB, angiotensin II receptor blocker; IRMA 2, Irbesartan Microalbuminuria Type 2 [study].

Progression of diabetic nephropathy in IRMA 2 study of hypertensive patients with type 2 diabetes and microproteinuria. Placebo represents medications other than an ARB or ACE inhibitor. In the irbesartan 150-mg and 300-mg groups, a medication other than another ARB or ACE inhibitor was added. The difference between placebo and 150 mg irbesartan was not significant ($P = 0.08$); between placebo and 300 mg irbesartan, $P <0.001$.

Parving HH, et al. *N Engl J Med*. 2001;345:875.

Overview of Completed Trials

In all three of the preceding trials, the ARB used was well tolerated. The results of these studies have important treatment implications and suggest that recommendations for treatment of hypertension in type 2 diabetics now include the use of ARBs as one of the preferred therapies. One of the trials (IDNT) indicated that renal disease progression can be delayed to a greater extent with an ARB than with a CCB (amlodipine)-based treatment program. In all cases, however, multiple medications will usually be necessary to achieve goal BPs—treatment should include the use of a diuretic. It is of interest to note that benefit in these studies occurred without a significant BP difference between groups of patients.

Data indicate that not only can the progression to more severe renal disease be slowed by the use of an ARB, but signs of glomerular dysfunction (ie, proteinuria) may be improved with a decrease in microproteinuria. These findings are similar to those regarding LVH in hypertension. LVH can be regressed with treatment or actually prevented if BP is lowered in hypertensive individuals before LVH becomes apparent.

Based on long-term trial evidence, the American Diabetes Association has noted that:

- In patients with type 2 diabetes, hypertension, and microalbuminuria, a regimen based on an ACE inhibitor or an ARB has been shown to delay the progression to macroalbuminuria
- In patients with type 2 diabetes, hypertension, macroalbuminuria (>300 mg/day), nephropathy, or renal insufficiency, an ARB should be strongly considered *as initial therapy*.

13

Recent Trials With ARBs

The Study on Cognition and Prognosis in the Elderly (SCOPE) trial recently reported results with the use of another ARB (candesartan), alone or in combination with other medications, on CV events as well as on cognitive function and quality of life in the elderly. In this double-blind, 4-year prospective study of almost 5000 elderly patients (ages 70 to 89 years), the group receiving candesartan plus other medications experienced a significant decrease in nonfatal stroke compared with patients on other medications. There was no significant difference in the occurrence of MI or CV mortality despite a greater decrease in BP in the candesartan-treated group. The study group showed less decline in speed of cognition than the control group over the period of the study, but no change in the working memory and some of the other functions tested. The investigators suggested that these findings may indicate that lowering BP with an ARB may be a useful strategy to delay or prevent dementia.

The Valsartan Antihypertensive Long-Term Use Evaluation (VALUE) prospective, randomized study comparing the effects of valsartan with those of amlodipine on CV morbidity and mortality in high-risk hypertensive patients is ongoing. Additional trials with ARBs are in progress and results of several other trials will be available within the next 2 to 3 years.

14 Calcium Channel Blockers

In the past 20 years, numerous calcium channel blockers (CCBs) have been introduced; a list of available CCBs appears in **Table 14**.**1**. The CCBs lower blood pressure (BP) by inhibiting the entry of calcium ions into vascular smooth muscle cells, which:

- Reduces vascular tone and contractility
- Results in vasodilation
- Reduces peripheral resistance
- Decreases BP.

There are several types of CCBs. The nondihydropyridines act on heart muscle as well as peripheral arterioles; they include (**Table 14**.**1**):

- Diltiazem
  - Cardizem CD
  - Cardizem LA
  - Dilacor XR
  - Tiazac
- Verapamil
  - Calan and Calan SR
  - Isoptin and Isoptin SR
  - Verelan PM
  - Covera-HS.

The dihydropyridine CCBs act primary on peripheral blood vessels; they include (**Table 14**.**1**):

- Amlodipine (Norvasc)
- Isradipine (DynCirc CR)
- Nisoldipine (Sular)
- Felodipine (Plendil).

14

TABLE 14.1 — CALCIUM CHANNEL BLOCKERS USED IN TREATING HYPERTENSION

Generic (Trade) Name	Usual Dosage Range		Physiologic Effects	Comments and Probable Side Effects
	Dose (mg)	Frequency		
Nondihydropyridines				
Diltiazem XR (Cardizem LA)	120-540	1/day	Block inward movement of calcium ions across cell membranes and cause smooth-muscle relaxation. Peripheral resistance ↓; BP ↓; heart rate ↔↓	Block slow channels in heart and may reduce sinus rate; increase degree of arteriovenous block; constipation
Diltiazem XR (Cardizem CD Dilacor XR, Tiazac)	180-420	1/day		
Verapamil IM (Calan, Isoptin)	80-320	2/day		
Verapamil LA (Calan SR, Isoptin SR)	120-360	1-2/day		
Verapamil-coer (Covera HS, Verelan PM)	120-360	1		

Dihydropyridines				
Amlodipine (Norvasc)	2.5-10	1/day	Block inward movement of calcium ion across cell membranes and cause smooth-muscle relaxation peripheral resistance ↓; BP ↓; heart rate ↔↑	More potent peripheral vasodilators than diltiazem and verapamil, but may cause more dizziness, headache, flushing, peripheral edema, and tachycardia
Felodipine (Plendil)	2.5-20	1/day		
Isradipine (DynaCirc CR)	2.5-10	2/day		
Nicardipine SR (Cardene SR)	60-120	2/day		
Nifedipine LA (Procardia XL, Adalat CC)	30-60	1/day		
Nisoldipine (Sular)	10-40	1/day		
Abbreviation: BP, blood pressure.				

14

Some CCBs, especially the verapamil type, may result in partial blockade of the atrioventricular (AV) or sinoatrial (SA) node, as well as have a negative inotropic effect. Sinus rate may be slowed and degree of heart block increased.

Nondihydropyridine Calcium Channel Blockers

In addition to lowering BP, the nondihydropyridine CCBs may be useful in the treatment of cardiac arrhythmias, especially in the treatment of supraventricular arrhythmias. Because of negative inotropic effects, however, left ventricular systolic function may be adversely affected and congestive heart failure (CHF) may result in some patients with ischemic heart disease. This is uncommon but is more likely to occur if this type of CCB is given in combination with a β-blocker. The long-acting formulations of diltiazem and verapamil are probably effective when given on a once-a-day basis. Currently, the shorter-acting formulations of diltiazem and verapamil are not recommended for therapy.

Dihydropyridine Calcium Channel Blockers

The dihydropyridine CCBs, such as nifedipine, nicardipine, isradipine, amlodipine, nisoldipine, and felodipine act primarily on peripheral vascular beds and have little effect on cardiac muscle contraction or AV conduction. They are probably effective given on a once-a-day basis. Short-acting dihydropyridine CCBs (eg, nifedipine) (**Table 14.1**) should probably not be used in the treatment of hypertension, despite the fact that they reduce BP. The short duration of BP lowering may result in reflux tachycardia and may contribute to an increase, not a decrease, in ischemic heart disease events.

CCBs are as effective in reducing BP as the other classes of drugs currently recommended as initial or alternative first-step therapy in the management of hypertension. Several studies suggest that a long-acting dihydropyridine (amlodipine) will reduce systolic blood pressure (SBP) to a greater extent than an angiotensin-converting enzyme (ACE) inhibitor. One study suggests that the percentage of patients achieving a target goal of diastolic blood pressure (DBP) reduction may be somewhat higher with diltiazem than with other drugs. The CCBs are as effective as diuretics in the elderly and in black patients, and are usually more effective than β-adrenergic inhibitors or ACE inhibitors in these individuals. In the Antihypertensive and Lipid-Lowering Treatment to Prevent Heart Attack Trial (ALLHAT), amlodipine reduced SBP by 0.8 mm Hg less and DBP 0.7 mm Hg more than chlorthalidone.

CCBs are effective as monotherapy in reducing BP in stage 1 and stage 2 hypertension; approximately 45% to 50% of patients will respond. As with other drugs, about 75% to 80% of hypertensive patients will become normotensive when a diuretic and a CCB are given together. For example, in one study, >50% of patients resistant to diltiazem became normotensive when a thiazide was added; >50% of patients resistant to a thiazide responded when diltiazem was added. A single combination pill of a CCB and a diuretic is not currently available and there are still some investigators who do not believe that the use of these two agents together is a useful combination. Despite the fact that CCBs may lower BP, in a large number of patients (including elderly and black individuals), outcome may not be as favorable as with other medications. Comparative studies with an ACE inhibitor and long-acting dihydropyridine CCBs in non–insulin-de-

14

pendent (type 2) diabetes and in the elderly indicate that patients in the ACE-inhibitor group experienced fewer fatal and nonfatal cardiovascular (CV) events (see below). In ALLHAT, however, the primary end points of fatal and nonfatal CHD events were similar with a CCB (amlodipine), an ACE inhibitor (lisinopril), and chlorthalidone, but the occurrence of heart failure was greater with the CCB than with the diuretic.

Several combination CCBs and ACE inhibitors have been approved for use. These combinations are also highly effective in lowering BP; when an ACE inhibitor is given with a dihydropyridine, the degree of edema is decreased and the degree of BP lowering and response rates are increased. Several studies in addition to ALLHAT have answered the question as to whether the use of CCBs will reduce morbidity and mortality in hypertensive patients. These studies provide information about the long-term effects on both cerebrovascular and CV morbidity and mortality when CCBs are used as baseline therapy (see below).

Syst Eur Trial

In the Systolic Hypertension in Europe (Syst Eur) randomized, placebo-controlled, blinded trial in elderly subjects, primarily with isolated systolic hypertension (ISH) defined as >160/<95 mm Hg, nitrendipine, a moderately long-acting dihydropyridine (not available in the United States), was used as initial therapy. The study was discontinued after about 2 years because of a significant reduction in fatal and nonfatal strokes in the treated compared with the placebo group. While there was a trend toward a reduction in coronary heart disease (CHD) events and heart failure, this did not achieve statistical significance. It is possible that this would have occurred if the study had continued for a longer period of time. Diabetic patients experienced an even greater benefit than nondiabetic subjects in this study. These results were similar to those noted in another trial in elderly patients with ISH (the Systolic Hypertension in the Elderly Program [SHEP] trial, which was diuretic based). Additional reductions in both fatal and nonfatal CV end points were noted when other medications (enalapril and/or hydrochlorothiazide) were added to nitrendipine therapy to achieve better BP control. Benefit in this trial was noted within the first 6 months of the study, an important point in considering the rationale for treating elderly hypertensive individuals. A reduction in CV events may occur within a short period of time if BP is lowered. An important finding was a reduction in the occurrence of dementia in this trial. As noted in Chapter 13, *Angiotensin II Receptor Blockers*, a slowing down of memory loss was noted in the Study on Cognition and Prognosis in the Elderly (SCOPE) trial with an angiotensin II receptor blocker (ARB).

In the 5-year diuretic-based SHEP study in the United States, both cerebrovascular and CV events were also significantly reduced (**Table 17.4**). On the basis of the SHEP and the Syst Eur trial results, a long-acting dihydropyridine may be appropriate therapy in an elderly patient with ISH if a diuretic is ineffective or poorly tolerated. This appears to be a reasonable recommendation.

As noted, the World Health Organization–International Society of Hypertension (WHO-ISH) and the European Societies of Hypertension and Cardiology reports suggested that CCBs could be used as initial monotherapy in patients of any age based on analyses that indicate a similar result with these agents and other medications if BP is reduced.

HOT Trial

The Hypertension Optimal Treatment (HOT) trial provides additional assurance that a long-acting dihydropyridine-based treatment program does not increase cardiac events. This was a concern based on some data with the shorter-acting CCBs (see *Effects on Coronary Heart Disease,* this chapter). The HOT trial used felodipine (a long-acting CCB) as baseline therapy with five titration stops (**Table 14.2**). Groups of patients were divided into three target BP cohorts: <90 mm Hg, <85 mm Hg, <80 mm Hg. Achieved BP differences at the end of the trial were minimal in the three groups. There were no significant differences in CV events among the three groups who achieved DBPs of 85, 83, and 81 mm Hg except among diabetics. Individuals who achieved the lowest BPs felt better than those at higher levels—a finding also noted in other trials. Perhaps hypertension is not always "silent." Some patients do have symptoms, especially vague headaches.

The study did not provide convincing evidence that lowering BP <135-140/80-85 mm Hg reduces CV events; on the other hand, lowering BP below this level did not appear to be harmful. It confirmed the importance of intensive BP lowering in diabetic subjects (**Table 14.3**) where the patients in the group with DBP of <80 mm Hg had fewer events than those in the <90 mm Hg target group. Events were reduced to a greater degree than previously reported in other clinical trials in all groups of patients, primarily, in this author's opinion, because of the careful attention paid to achieving lower BP. Whereas in other trials as many as 20% to 30% of subjects failed to achieve even a DBP of <90 mm Hg, only 8% remained above this level in the HOT study.

As noted, the tight BP control study in type 2 diabetics (United Kingdom Prospective Diabetes Study [UKPDS] 38) has also emphasized the importance of good BP control in diabetics. In this study, an achieved BP of 144/82 mm Hg compared with 154/87 mm Hg in a group that was not as well controlled resulted in

TABLE 14.2 — THE HYPERTENSION OPTIMAL TREATMENT (HOT) TRIAL

Patient Demographics	Therapy	End of Study	Achieved BP in the Three Target Groups (mm Hg)
• No. of patients: 18,790 • Average age: 61.5 years • Mean SBP: 170 mm Hg • Mean DBP: 105 mm Hg	Step 1: Felodipine 5 mg qd (CCB) Step 2: ACE inhibitor or β-blocker added Step 3: Dosage titration with CCB Step 4: Dosage titration with ACE inhibitor or β-blocker Step 5: Add a diuretic	• 78% on CCB • 41% on ACE inhibitor • 28% on β-blocker • 22% on diuretic	• DBP <90 = 144/85 • DBP <85 = 141/83 • DBP <80 = 140/81

Abbreviations: ACE, angiotensin-converting enzyme; CCB, calcium channel blocker; DBP, diastolic blood pressure; SBP, systolic blood pressure.

14

TABLE 14.3 — SUMMARY OF THE HYPERTENSION OPTIMAL TREATMENT (HOT) TRIAL

- No significant different in cardiovascular (CV) events or total mortality in subjects with achieved target diastolic blood pressures (DBPs) of 85, 83, or 81 mm Hg
- Most of the benefit achieved with BP levels of <140/85-90 mm Hg
- Overall event rate lower than in previous studies, probably because of pronounced lowering of BP (only 8.5% of subjects ended with DBP >90 mm Hg compared with about 20% to 30% in previous trials)
- In patients with diabetes mellitus:
  – *Major CV events and CV mortality* reduced significantly greater in target group (<80 mm Hg compared to <90 mm Hg)
  – No significant difference in stroke, all myocardial infarction (MI), or total mortality
- In patients with ischemic heart disease: no significant difference in major CV events between target groups with DBPs <90, <85, and <80 mm Hg

a statistically significant reduction in CV events. This was probably the result of better BP control and not specific therapy since there was no difference in outcome between a β-blocker–based and an ACE inhibitor–based program. Many patients in the study required multiple drugs to achieve goal BP.

Recommendations of many national committees and the American Diabetes Association reflect the results of these trials: *target BP in diabetic patients should be set lower than the goal of <140/90 mm Hg for other patients; and combination therapy with different classes of medications is most often necessary to lower BP to goal levels of <130/80-85 mm Hg.*

The HOT study also demonstrated that the use of aspirin 75 mg/day in hypertensive patients decreased all myocardial infarctions (MIs) and major CV events. No effect was noted on stroke, CV, or total mortality.

There was an increase in nonserious gum and gastrointestinal bleeding. These are important observations; aspirin can be given in small doses to hypertensive subjects with the expectation of benefit *if BP is controlled.*

Adverse Reactions

Side effects differ considerably among the various CCBs. This is not unexpected, given their different sites of action. The dihydropyridine derivatives, especially the shorter-acting preparations, may cause:

- Flushing
- Headache
- Postural dizziness
- Palpitations or tachycardia
- Ankle edcma.

The shorter-acting preparations should be used with caution or not at all in the treatment of hypertension.

The longer-acting CCBs, such as nisoldipine and amlodipine, and longer-acting formulations of nifedipine (Procardia XL), isradipine (DynaCirc CR), etc, cause fewer side effects than the shorter-acting derivatives. Although some studies suggest that reflex tachycardia is not common, an increase in heart rate may occur even with these medications. Ankle edema is a concern to patients who are used to being warned about ankle swelling as a sign of CHF. Swelling may occur with small doses of any of these compounds and may not respond to diuretics although this may occur in some cases. Edema results from the seepage of fluid from the capillary bed as a result of vasodilation. It usually clears with bed rest.

Verapamil may cause severe constipation, postural hypotension, headache, and dizziness, and may have a negative inotropic effect on cardiac muscle contraction. Diltiazem may cause headache and some GI disturbances. CCBs have not been shown to have any adverse effects on lipid metabolism or on insulin sensitivity. There is no evidence of any renal function deterioration when these drugs are used.

Effects on Coronary Heart Disease

To date, studies with the dihydropyridine CCBs have not shown a significant benefit in preventing a recurrence of MI in patients with ischemic heart disease. The rate of reinfarction does appear to be decreased in patients with ischemic heart disease when verapamil or diltiazem is used, but overall mortality is not reduced. Some data suggest that the incidence of MI may actually be increased when a short-acting dihydropyridine CCB such as nifedipine is used in hypertensive subjects. As noted, these agents should be used with caution or not at all in the management of hypertension.

Comparative Trials in Hypertension

There have been several important comparative trials with CCBs:

- A 3-year study that compared a diuretic (hydrochlorothiazide) and a shorter-acting formulation of a dihydropyridine CCB (isradipine) reported a greater incidence of CV events in the CCB group, primarily new-onset angina.
- In another 2-year study, Verapamil in Hypertension Atherosclerosis Study (VHAS) where a long-acting formulation of verapamil SR (240 mg/day) was compared with chlorthalidone (25 mg/day), a similar degree of BP lowering occurred, –28/–17 mm Hg and –29/–17 mm Hg, respectively. No differences in adverse events were recorded and the number of fatal and non-

fatal CV events were similar in the two groups. This study indicated that a longer-acting formulation of a nondihydropyridine CCB was safe and did not cause an increase in CV events; on the other hand, it did not appear to be more effective than a diuretic.

- Several long-term comparative 4- to 5-year morbidity/mortality trials based on CCB-treatment programs have been completed. Both the International Nifedipine Gastrointestinal Therapeutic System Study Intervention as a Goal for Hypertension Therapy (INSIGHT) and the Nordic Diltiazem (NORDIL) trials have reported that *overall* cardiac events were similar with the use of a CCB-based treatment program and a diuretic/potassium-sparing medication–based program (INSIGHT) or a β-blocker/diuretic–based treatment program (NORDIL). In both of these studies, a high percentage of subjects received multiple medications. The majority of subjects were >60 years of age. BP reduction in the INSIGHT study was from baseline levels of 173/99 mm Hg to 138/82 mm Hg, with little difference between the two treatment groups, ie, nifedipine and diuretic. In the NORDIL study, BP decreased from 174/106 mm Hg to 152/88 mm Hg in the diltiazem group and to 149/87 mm Hg in the diuretic/β-blocker group.

- A recent trial, the International Verapamil SR/Trandolapril Study (INVEST), evaluated the occurrence of CV disease end points in 22,000 patients with hypertension and CHD. A regimen based on the use of sustained-release verapamil (with an ACE inhibitor [trandolapril] and a diuretic added if necessary) was compared with a treatment program based on atenolol with a thiazide or ACE inhibitor added. Target SBP of

14

<140 mm Hg for nondiabetics and <130 mm Hg for diabetics or patients with renal disease were achieved in 64% of patients; goal DBP of <90 and <85 mm Hg, respectively, were achieved in 91% in both groups. No differences in BP or outcome from CV death, MI, or nonfatal stroke were noted between the two groups. More than 80% of patients required more than one drug to control BP. Of interest is that only 6.16% of patients in the verapamil group developed new-onset diabetes compared with 7.2% in the atenolol group (12% to 13% difference) (**Table 13.3**).

As noted, overall end points in these studies were essentially similar regardless of the medications used (**Tables 14.4 and 14.5**). *But* there were some differences: fewer strokes with diltiazem in the NORDIL study, fewer fatal MIs and CHF with diuretics in the INSIGHT trial. The total number of events was small. Results of the ALLHAT trial indicate that fatal MI rates were similar with a long-acting dihydropyridine (amlodipine) and a diuretic. On the other hand, they are consistent with the INSIGHT data that the occurrence of CHF may be greater with a CCB. These differences may disappear if a diuretic is used with the CCB. The INVEST results in patients with CHD indicate that results in a CCB-based trial (with an ACE inhibitor) are equivalent to those with a β-blocker/diuretic–based regimen but with fewer incidences of new-onset diabetes in the CCB/ACE inhibitor group.

Adverse reactions (side effects) were similar in the NORDIL study between diltiazem and the diuretic/β-blocker groups, but in the INSIGHT (nifedipine) study, side effects (ie, peripheral edema and headache) occurred in >10% of subjects and were more common with nifedipine than with the diuretic/potassium-sparing group.

TABLE 14.4 — INSIGHT STUDY*: CARDIOVASCULAR EVENTS		
	Nifedipine	Co-Amiloride
Primary end points	200 (6.3%)	182 (5.8%)
Myocardial infarctions		
Fatal	16 (0.5%)	5 (0.2%)[†]
Nonfatal	61 (1.9%)	56 (1.8%)
Strokes		
Fatal	55 (1.7%)	63 (2.0%)
Nonfatal	12 (0.3%)	11 (0.3%)
Heart failure	24 (0.8%)	11 (0.3%)[†]

Abbreviation: INSIGHT, International Nifedipine Gastrointestinal Therapeutic System Study Intervention as a Goal for Hypertension Therapy.

No difference in overall primary end points (cardiovascular morbidity and mortality) between nifedipine and a diuretic. A significant difference was noted, however, in the occurrence of fatal myocardial infarctions and congestive heart failure—fewer events occurred with the diuretic.

* Total number of patients studied: 6321.
† Statistically significant difference.

Results from the African American Study of Kidney Disease (AASK) trial indicate that the use of an ACE inhibitor (ramipril)–based or a β-blocker (metoprolol)– based treatment program in black patients results in less progression of renal disease in patients with significant proteinuria (>1 g/day) than the use of a long-acting dihydropyridine (amlodipine). In this trial, results were significantly better with the ACE inhibitor than with other therapies.

TABLE 14.5 — NORDIL STUDY*: NUMBER OF PATIENTS WITH EVENTS PER 1000 PATIENT-YEARS

Event	Number of Patients Studied (Events Per 1000 Patient Years)	
	Diltiazem	Diuretics/ β-Blockers
Primary end points[†]	403 (16.6)	400 (16.2)
All strokes	159 (6.4)	196 (7.9)[‡]
Myocardial infarctions	183 (7.4)	157 (6.3)
Cardiovascular death	131 (5.2)	115 (4.5)
Congestive heart failure	63 (2.5)	53 (2.1)

Abbreviation: NORDIL, Nordic Diltiazem Study.

Strokes were more common in the diuretics/β-blocker group, but a nonsignificant trend toward higher levels of myocardial infarction, cardiovascular death, and congestive heart failure was noted in the diltiazem group.

* Total number of patients studied: 10,881.
† All strokes, myocardial infarctions, and other cardiovascular deaths.
‡ Statistically significant

Summary: Where Do the Calcium Channel Blockers Fit in a Treatment Program?

The CCBs are effective antihypertensive agents that are generally well tolerated. Some data suggest that these drugs (usually in combination with other agents) may be as, but not more, effective in reducing morbidity and mortality in hypertensive subjects when compared with other agents, ie, diuretics or β-blockers. CCBs are considerably more costly than those medications. Some data suggest that ACE inhibitors may reduce CV events, especially MI and heart failure, to a greater degree than CCBs in the elderly and in patients with diabetes and that either ACE inhibitors or β-blockers are probably better choices in hypertensive patients with renal disease and proteinuria or ischemic heart disease.

The Seventh Joint National Committee (JNC 7) on the Prevention, Detection, Evaluation, and Treatment of High Blood Pressure suggests that an ACE inhibitor or an ARB should be one of the preferred medications in patients with diabetes and renal disease. In ISH, a CCB can be used if a diuretic is ineffective or poorly tolerated. In many situations, a CCB can be used in combination with another agent (ie, a diuretic, an ACE inhibitor, an ARB or in the case of the dihydropyridines, a β-blocker) to achieve goal BP. There are many instances when the addition of a CCB to a treatment program in a patient who has not responded will result in the achievement of goal BP. Currently, these agents should probably not be considered initial therapy for most patients unless there are specific contraindications for the use of other drugs or specific indications for their use (**Table 4.5**). Better results will probably be obtained with these agents if they are used more frequently with diuretics. Studies are under way to evaluate CCB/diuretic combinations.

15 Approach to Treatment: Combination Therapy

In the 1950s, the treatment of hypertension was fairly simple. The only drugs that had been proved useful and relatively safe were reserpine, hydralazine, and diuretics. Others, such as the veratrum derivatives and the ganglion-blocking drugs, lowered blood pressure (BP) but presented unacceptable side effects in a high percentage of patients. Choices for therapy became more difficult when α-methyldopa, the β-adrenergic inhibitors, peripheral adrenergic inhibitors (eg, guanethidine), and the centrally acting drugs (such as clonidine) became available; results of therapy were not always satisfactory.

In the past 20 years, treatment has greatly improved with the availability of α_1-receptor blockers, α_1- and β-blockers, angiotensin-converting enzyme (ACE) inhibitors, calcium channel blockers (CCBs), angiotensin II receptor blockers (ARBs), and, most recently, a better tolerated aldosterone antagonist; but choosing the appropriate therapy may present a problem for many physicians. We believe, however, that a simple approach can still be taken in the majority of patients.

There is some rationale for using a type of **15** stepped-care management, although not necessarily the type of stepped-care advocated in 1977 by the First Joint National Committee (JNC-I) on Detection, Evaluation, and Treatment of High Blood Pressure. Dr. Irvine Page, one of the pioneers in hypertension research, once commented that "stepped-care is merely an attempt to bring order out of chaos." We agree. Stepped-care implies that if BP is not reduced to normal with one drug, it is appropriate to add small doses of another drug from another class. Not all experts concur with this approach, and some still favor using a sequence of different medications, one at time—if the first is ineffective, discontinue it and try another, and so on. Our reasons for not favoring this method of therapy are presented below.

The JNC-VI report issued in 1997 suggested that initial monotherapy should include the use of either a diuretic or a β-adrenergic inhibitor unless there are specific indications for another medication. This recommendation is similar to that of JNC-V in 1993. It was not based on the fact that these drugs are necessarily more effective in reducing BP than other medications, but rather, at the time of the report, that they were the only drugs that had been tested and shown in clinical trials with hypertensive individuals to reduce cerebrovascular and cardiovascular (CV) morbidity and mortality. Since that time, numerous long-term outcome trials that utilized ACE inhibitors, CCBs, or ARBs and comparative trials of different agents have been published. These have been reviewed.

Some modifications in recommendations for specific drug therapy have been suggested based on reports of newer studies, including:

- Verapamil in Hypertension Atherosclerosis Study (VHAS)
- Hypertension Optimal Treatment (HOT)
- Captopril Prevention Project (CAPPP)
- United Kingdom Prospective Diabetes Study (UKPDS)
- Swedish Trial in Old Persons With Hypertension 2 (STOP-Hypertension-2)
- Nordic Diltiazem (NORDIL) study
- Appropriate Blood Pressure Control in Diabetes (ABCD)
- Fosinopril Versus Amlodipine Cardiovascular Events Trial (FACET)

- African American Study of Kidney Disease and Hypertension (AASK)
- International Nifedipine Gastrointestinal Therapeutic System Study Intervention as a Goal for Hypertension Therapy (INSIGHT)
- Reduction in Endpoints in Patients With Non–Insulin-Dependent Diabetes Mellitus With the Angiotensin II Antagonist Losartan (RENAAL)
- Irbesartan Diabetic Nephropathy Trial (IDNT)
- Irbesartan Microalbuminuria Type 2 Diabetes Mellitus in Hypertension Patients (IRMA 2)
- Losartan Intervention for End-Point Reduction in Hypertension (LIFE) study
- Antihypertensive and Lipid-Lowering Treatment to Prevent Heart Attack Trial (ALLHAT)
- Australian National Blood Pressure (ANBP 2) study
- Study on Cognition and Prognosis in the Elderly (SCOPE)
- Controlled Onset Verapamil Investigation of Cardiovascular End Points (CONVINCE) trial.
- International Verapamil SR/Trandolapril Study (INVEST).

The JNC 7 has incorporated the results of these studies in their recommendations. Most of the newer data indicate that results with CCBs and ACE inhibitors are equal to but no better than those with diuretics or diuretics/β-blockers, and that the use of a diuretic-based regimen is more effective in reducing congestive heart failure (CHF) events than a CCB. The ALLHAT results suggest that a diuretic may be more effective in reducing stroke or overall CV events than an ACE inhibitor. However, as noted, coronary heart disease (CHD)–event results were similar with the diuretic, ACE inhibitor, and CCB in ALLHAT. In most instances, the degree of BP lowering appears to be more important

15

than the specific medications used to achieve it. There are, however, some exceptions (ie, ACE inhibitors appear to be more beneficial than CCBs in reducing myocardial infarction [MI]), heart failure, and progression of renal disease; α-blockers are less effective than diuretics). A regimen that includes an ACE inhibitor or an ARB appears to reduce the occurrence of new-onset diabetes compared with a treatment program that does not include one of these agents (**Table 13**.3).

In general, however, the use of a diuretic alone or in combination with other medications should remain the initial choice for therapy with some caveats that have been discussed. The choice of an ACE inhibitor, an ARB, a β-blocker, or a CCB (usually with a diuretic) is also acceptable as initial therapy. ARBs have been recommended by the American Diabetes Association as initial therapy in diabetics, especially those with evidence of nephropathy; but, in most cases, a diuretic has to be used to achieve goal BP (see Chapter 4, *Drug Treatment of Hypertension: General Information, Specific Drug Therapy* section; and **Table 4**.3, **Table 15**.1, **Table 15**.2, **Table 15**.3, and **Table 15**.4). **Table 15**.2 is from JNC 7 and reflects newer data.

TABLE 15.1 — CHARACTERISTICS OF AN IDEAL STEP-1 DRUG

- Use as monotherapy—results in normotensive blood pressure levels in a high percentage of cases
- Long-acting—simple titration to an effective dose
- Few subjective side effects
- Few adverse metabolic effects
- Blood pressure–lowering effects do not disappear over time
- There is a decrease in morbidity and mortality following its use
- Relatively inexpensive

Characteristics of an Ideal Medication for Initial Therapy

Almost all of the available medications satisfy many or most of the criteria of an ideal antihypertensive agent (**Table 15.1**):

- Most are effective as monotherapy in about 40% to 60% of patients.
- Most can be given on a once-a-day basis with few visits for titration.
- Other than the centrally acting drugs and perhaps some of the α_1-blockers, side effects are not a major problem in the majority of patients. Side effects can be minimized by starting with small doses.
- Although the use of diuretics and β-blockers may result in some change in lipid levels, these are usually short term in the case of diuretics and are of doubtful clinical significance with the β-blockers. The clinical significance of these changes has been overemphasized. It also does not appear at present that the effects of diuretics on insulin resistance are clinically important.
- Long-term effectiveness in lowering BP has been proven with most available antihypertensive drugs, and extensive old and newer data suggest a reduction in both cerebrovascular and CV morbidity and mortality when a diuretic-, β-blocker–, ACE inhibitor–, or CCB-based regimen is used. More recent data with ARBs also indicate that these agents are effective in reducing renal disease progression, especially in diabetics, and suggest that a regimen based on ARBs may also reduce overall CV events and stroke when compared with a β-blocker regimen in hypertensive patients with left ventricular hypertrophy (LVH). Most studies used com-

15

TABLE 15.2 — SPECIFIC INDICATIONS AND CONTRAINDICATIONS FOR PARTICULAR ANTIHYPERTENSIVE DRUGS*

Clinical Situation	May Have Favorable Effects	Requires Careful Follow-Up	Contraindicated
Cardiovascular			
Angina pectoris	β-Blockers, CCBs	—	Direct vasodilators
Bradycardia/heart block, sick sinus syndrome	—	—	β-Blockers, labetalol, verapamil, diltiazem
Cardiac failure—systolic dysfunction	Diuretics, ACE inhibitors, ARBs, α_1–β-blockers (carvedilol), some β-blockers, aldosterone antagonists	—	Calcium channel blockers
Hypertrophic cardiomyopathy with diastolic dysfunction	β-Blockers, diltiazem, verapamil, α_1–β-blockers (carvedilol)	Diuretics	α_1-Blockers, hydralazine, minoxidil
Hyperdynamic circulation (rapid heart rate)	β-Blockers	—	Direct vasodilators
Peripheral vascular occlusive disease	—	β-Blockers	—
After myocardial infarction	Non-ISA β-blockers, ACE inhibitors (selected patients), verapamil, or diltiazem	—	Direct vasodilators

Renal		
Bilateral renal arterial disease or severe stenosis of artery to solitary kidney	—	ACE inhibitors, ARBs
Renal insufficiency: early (serum creatinine 1.5-2.5 mg/dL)	—	Potassium-sparing agents, potassium supplements
Advanced (serum creatinine ≥2.5-3.0 mg/dL)	Loop diuretics	ACE inhibitors, diuretics, ARBs	Potassium-sparing agents, potassium supplements
Depression	α_2-Agonists	Reserpine
Diabetes mellitus–type 1 (insulin-dependent)	ACE inhibitor or possibly ARBs with a diuretic	β-Blockers	—
Diabetes mellitus–type 2 (with or without proteinemia)	ACE inhibitor or ARBs usually with a diuretic, β-blocker/diuretic	Use with caution in patients with serum creatinine >3 mg/dL	—
Liver disease	—	Labetalol	Methyldopa
Vascular headache (migraine)	β-Blockers, nondihydropyridine CCBs	—	—

Abbreviations: ACE, angiotensin-converting enzyme; ARB, angiotensin II receptor blocker; CCB, calcium channel blocker; ISA, intrinsic sympathomimetic activity.

* Not all indications or contraindications are listed. See also Tables 15.3 and 15.4.

15

TABLE 15.3 — SPECIFIC INDICATIONS AND CONTRAINDICATIONS FOR PARTICULAR ANTIHYPERTENSIVE DRUGS IN PREGNANCY*

Clinical Situation	Indicated	Requires Careful Follow-up	Contraindicated
Pregnancy			
Preeclampsia	Methyldopa, hydralazine	—	ACE inhibitors, ARBs
Chronic hypertension	Same medications as prior to pregnancy except for ACE inhibitors or ARBs	—	ACE inhibitors, ARBs

Abbreviations: ACE, angiotensin-converting enzyme; ARB, angiotensin II receptor blocker.

* Not all indications or contraindications are listed. See also Tables 15.2 and 15.4.

binations of two or three different agents. Longer-acting CCB-based treatment programs result in essentially similar overall outcomes on CV morbidity and mortality as with a diuretic/β-blocker–based program except for some differences in two studies in the occurrence of CHF and MI where diuretics proved to be more beneficial. In the STOP-Hypertension-2, ACE-inhibitor treatment proved superior to CCB therapy in the elderly, and as repeatedly emphasized, several smaller studies suggest that fewer episodes of CHF or MI occur in an ACE inhibitor–based treatment program than in a CCB-based program in patients with diabetes. As noted, in the ALLHAT, the occurrence of CHD events was similar with a CCB, an ACE inhibitor, and a thiazide diuretic, but heart failure was more frequent with a CCB than with a diuretic.

- In the initial choice of drug, cost should be considered. It has been reported that as many as 20% to 25% of patients are unable to afford to fill their prescriptions. It is foolhardy to recommend a drug if the patient is unable to afford it. The class of drug, recommended as step-1 therapy by JNC 7, happens to be the least expensive; but many of the other drugs, such as ACE inhibitors or CCBs, are now available at lower cost than several years ago. *If ongoing studies demonstrate that a more expensive medication is more effective than a less costly one, then cost should be a secondary issue.* However, since recent studies suggest that the more-expensive agents do not reduce morbidity and mortality to a greater extent than less-expensive agents, then cost becomes an important consideration in the choice of treatment.

15

TABLE 15.4 — INDICATIONS AND CONTRAINDICATIONS FOR INITIAL MONOTHERAPY WITH ANTIHYPERTENSIVE MEDICATIONS*

ACE Inhibitors and Angiotensin II Receptor Blockers
- Not as effective in blacks as monotherapy.
- Avoid in patients with bilateral renal artery stenosis and in pregnant women.
- Especially useful in congestive heart failure when added to a diuretic and/or digitalis.
- Although some investigators have suggested that ACE inhibitors are not as effective as diuretics in the elderly, there is evidence that both classes of drugs will lower blood pressure and reduce morbidity and mortality in this group of patients.
- May be especially effective in diabetics or diabetic nephropathy (usually with a diuretic to bring blood pressure levels down to goal levels of <130-135/85 mm Hg).

α_1-Blockers
- Useful in men with prostatic hypertrophy.

β-Blockers
- Less effective in blacks (may be more effective than diuretics in whites); α_1-β-blockers are effective in both black and white populations.
- Avoid in patients with a history of asthma, chronic obstructive pulmonary disease, or with definite evidence of peripheral arterial disease, marked bradycardia, and possibly in insulin-dependent diabetics. (Compounds with intrinsic sympathomimetic activity may not cause bradycardia.)
- Especially useful in patients with angina.
- The α_1-β-blocker carvedilol and some β-blockers are useful in congestive heart failure.
- Especially useful in patients with migraine.

Calcium Channel Blockers
- Effective in lowering blood pressure in both black and white patients, and in young and elderly patients.
- Useful in patients with angina.

Diuretics
- Effective in lowering blood pressure in both black and white patients, and in young and elderly patients.
- Probably should not be used in patients with a history of gout.
- Thiazide diuretics are less effective as antihypertensive agents in the presence of renal insufficiency (>2.5 mg/dL creatinine). In these instances, a loop diuretic (ie, furosemide, bumetanide, torsemide) or metolazone should be used, probably in combination with other medications.
- May have favorable effect on osteoporosis.
- Morbidity and mortality outcome data continue to indicate that these agents should be part of most treatment programs.

Abbreviation: ACE, angiotensin-converting enzyme.

* Not all indications and contraindications are listed. See also Tables 15.2 and 15.3.

Factors Influencing the Choice of Initial Therapy

The type of treatment program that we prefer to follow considers certain demographic factors in selecting the initial drug. In general, a thiazide diuretic is the drug of choice for most patients. These are some differences in response that may be helpful:

- Whites and younger patients (<50 years of age) generally respond better to an adrenergic inhibitor such as a β-blocker, an ACE inhibitor, or an ARB. These patients also respond to a diuretic or a CCB, but the percentage of normotensive responders is somewhat lower.
- Blacks and older patients respond better to a diuretic or a CCB. Normotensive levels may also be achieved with a β-blocker, an ACE inhibitor, or an ARB, but a smaller percentage of patients become normotensive. The reason for

15

these differences has not been determined. It may or may not be related to pretreatment renin levels. Attempts to define potential responders by measuring plasma renin levels have not proved reliable in most instances.

These general guidelines can be helpful in selecting a step-1 drug. Other factors that are important include:

- If the patient has a concomitant disease, such as asthma, insulin-dependent diabetes, or definite peripheral arterial disease, a β-blocker usually should not be chosen.
- If a patient has a history of gout, it might be prudent to avoid a diuretic. If BP is not normalized with another medication, a diuretic can be added, but allopurinol may also be necessary to control uric acid levels.
- In patients who are very physically active, β-adrenergic inhibitors may not be a good first choice unless there are specific reasons for their use (eg, post-MI, angina, migraine headache).
- In patients with angina, a β-adrenergic inhibitor or a long-acting CCB may be preferred as initial therapy. But if the patient is hypertensive and goal BPs are not achieved, a diuretic should be added.
- In patients with CHF or diabetic nephropathy, an ACE inhibitor or an ARB (plus a diuretic) would be preferred. In view of recent data, these agents (along with a small dose of a diuretic) may also be considered as initial therapy in diabetic patients without evidence of nephropathy. An α_1–β-blocker (carvedilol) or certain β-blockers (ie, bisoprolol or metoprolol) should be considered in patients with CHF (in addition to usual therapy).

- In patients with a previous MI, a β-blocker without intrinsic sympathomimetic activity is preferred.
- Based on evidence (see Chapter 5, *Diuretics* and Chapter 6, β-*Adrenergic Receptor Blockers*), there is no reason to avoid the use of diuretics or β-blockers in patients with hyperlipidemia and/or hyperglycemia. Although β-blockers may increase triglycerides or reduce high-density lipoprotein (HDL) over the long term, these effects may not be of clinical importance. Chemical changes should be monitored and the drug discontinued or dosage decreased if significant changes occur.

All of the preceding discussion regarding initial therapy may be moot—many patients should be started on two different medications as initial therapy.

Tables 15.2, **15.3**, and **15.4** summarize some specific indications and cautions regarding the use of antihypertensive drugs. **Table 15.5** outlines characteristics of different antihypertensive medications.

The plan for initial medical therapy that we most often follow is shown in **Figure 15.1**. This is generally similar to the JNC 7 recommendations, with a few exceptions based on recent trial data and a long experience in the management of hypertension. A diuretic in small doses equivalent to 12.5 mg chlorthalidone or 12.5 mg to 25 mg hydrochlorothiazide (HCTZ) is given to most patients unless there is a specific contraindication to its use or a specific indication for the use of another agent (see above). A β-blocker, an ACE inhibitor, or an ARB is also an acceptable choice for initial therapy, although these agents may not be the best choices for elderly patients. The use of a long-

TABLE 15.5 — PHYSIOLOGIC CHARACTERISTICS OF DIFFERENT ANTIHYPERTENSIVE MEDICATIONS*

	ACE/ARBs	Diuretics†	β-Blockers	α₁-β-Blockers	CCBs	α₁-Blockers	Centrally Acting Agents	Vasodilators
Peripheral vascular resistance	↓	↓	↑↔	↓	↓	↓	↓	↓
Cardiac output	↔	↔	↓	↔	↔	↔	↔	↑
Heart rate	↔↑	↔	↓	↔	Variable	↑	↔	↑
Total cholesterol	↔	Short term ↑	↔	↔	↔	↓	↔	↔
LDL cholesterol	↔	Short term ↑	↔	↔	↔	↓	↔↓	↔
HDL cholesterol	↔	↔	↔↓	↔	↔	↔↑	↔↓	↔
Triglycerides	↔↓	↑	↑	↑	↔	↔↓	↔↑	↔
Race (black/white)	Less effective in blacks	Effective in both	Less effective in blacks	Effective in both	Effective in both	Effective in both	Probably effective in both	Effective in both

Abbreviations: ACE, angiotensin-converting enzyme; ARB, angiotensin II receptor blocker; CCB, calcium channel blocker.

* Most of the available medications reduce peripheral resistance.
† Adverse effects on lipid levels are short term with diuretics—effects on triglycerides and HDL levels with β-blockers are of questionable clinical significance.

FIGURE 15.1 — INITIAL PHARMACOLOGIC TREATMENT OF HYPERTENSION*

Lifestyle modifications → Not at goal blood pressure (<140/90 mm Hg); or even lower in diabetics or patients with renal disease

Initial Drug Choices†

Diuretics in most cases; other classes of drugs may also be used

In stage 2 hypertensive patients or stage 1 hypertensive patients with diabetes or coronary heart disease, a combination of two medications is appropriate as initial therapy‡ (diuretic/β-blocker, diuretic/ACE inhibitor, diuretic/ARB, or diuretic/CCB combinations)

Specific Drug Indications for the Following Conditions:

Heart failure ---------------- ACE inhibitors, diuretics, carvedilol, some β-blockers, ARBs, aldosterone antagonists

Diabetes mellitus, with or without proteinuria ---------------- ACE inhibitors, ARBs, or β-blockers with diuretic

Post-myocardial infarction ---------------- β-Blockers, ACE inhibitors

Isolated systolic hypertension ---------------- Diuretics (preferred), CCBs (alternative therapy) or combinations of small doses of two medications

Abbreviations: ACE, angiotensin-converting enzyme; ARB, angiotensin II receptor blocker; CCB, calcium channel blocker.

* Modified from JNC 7.
† Unless contraindicated.
‡ See text.

15

acting CCB is also a possibility if there are reasons not to use other medications. If some BP lowering is noted but normotensive levels are not achieved, the dose of the diuretic should be increased (ie, to 25 mg chlorthalidone or 37.5 mg HCTZ). A potassium-sparing thiazide combination (eg, Dyazide or Maxzide) or an aldosterone antagonist (eg, eplerenone) can be used with the thiazides, especially in elderly patients, diabetics, or patients receiving digitalis.

If goal BP levels of <140/90 mm Hg are not achieved with the diuretic alone, a second drug (ie, a β-adrenergic inhibitor, an ACE inhibitor, an ARB, or, in some cases, a long-acting CCB) can be added. If another medication was used as initial therapy, a diuretic should be added unless there is a contraindication to its use. Based upon extensive trial data, an ACE inhibitor or an ARB, usually with a small dose of a diuretic, is also acceptable initial therapy. As suggested by JNC 7, the two-medication approach is appropriate in patients with stage 2 hypertension or stage 1 hypertension with diabetes or CHD.

Despite findings from some trials that the use of a CCB results in an equivalent number of CV events to the use of a diuretic/β-blocker or an ACE inhibitor, the incidence of CHF and MI appears to be higher with the CCBs than with other medications. Based on these data, a CCB is probably not preferred, at least at present, as initial monotherapy.

In the situation where a patient has been started on an ACE inhibitor, an ARB, or a CCB as monotherapy, a diuretic should be added if normalization of BP has not occurred.

If no BP-lowering effect is noted with initial therapy or if troublesome side effects occur, the first medication should be discontinued and another agent substituted. This is relatively rare.

As noted elsewhere, the World Health Organization–International Society of Hypertension (WHO-

ISH) and the European Societies reports suggest a somewhat different approach to initial therapy. These guidelines suggest that any of the available medications may be used as initial treatment. While it does appear that in most instances the degree of BP lowering is more important than the manner in which it is achieved, there are exceptions. These have already been reviewed in detail:

- α_1-Blockers do not appear to be as effective as diuretics.
- Several studies suggest that an ACE-inhibitor–based program results in fewer CV events than a CCB program in the elderly and in diabetics despite similar decreases in BP.
- Data suggest that the use of a diuretic results in fewer episodes of MI and CHF than a long-acting CCB
- An ARB-based treatment program results in fewer strokes, a decrease in composite end points of CV death, MI, and stroke, and fewer cases of new onset diabetes than a β-blocker–based program in hypertensive patients with LVH.

Comments on this recommendation are noted in Chapter 4, *Drug Treatment of Hypertension: General Information*.

Multiple-Drug Therapy or Sequential Monotherapy?

15

Using small doses of two different classes of drugs makes good sense, rather than increasing the dosage of one drug to a maximum level. BP response is generally better; as noted, about 75% to 80% of patients will respond to a combination of two different agents, whereas only about 50% to 55% will respond even to full doses of one drug. In addition, certain homeostatic reflex mechanisms may be blocked and side effects minimized by this approach. For example, the use of a diuretic alone will result in increased activity of the renin-angiotensin system, which may possibly prevent the achievement of normotensive levels in some patients. The addition of an ACE inhibitor, an ARB, or a β-blocker will blunt this effect. Studies have shown that contrary to what some physicians believe, adverse reactions are less frequent with smaller doses of two different medications compared with larger doses of one medication. The JNC 7 recognizes these benefits of low-dose combination therapy and, as noted, suggests that this approach may be appropriate initial therapy in many patients.

With this approach, dosage adjustments and BP monitoring can be at 2- to 3-month intervals in stage 1 and, in some cases, stage 2 hypertension. In more severe cases or if medications produce adverse effects, office visits must obviously be more frequent. Once BP is controlled at normotensive levels, patients need be seen only two to three times a year.

On the other hand, *sequential monotherapy* involves the use of individual drugs, one at time. If one is not completely effective, it is discontinued and another medication tried. Although this method is expensive, requires more frequent office visits, and is time-consuming, it is advocated by some experts. One disadvantage is that when this type of program is followed, patients may get the feeling that the physician is not quite sure of what he or she is doing, ie, trying one drug, another drug 2 months later, and a third drug 2 months after that. Confidence in therapy is more easily gained if BP reduction is brought about fairly quickly, even if more than one medication has to be used.

If BPs have been normalized for about 1 year after initiating therapy, it is reasonable to consider reducing the dosage of the first drug (which might not have been effective) to see if the second drug can maintain normotensive levels. It could be argued that if the first drug was relatively ineffective, why not stop it? However, effects on BP of different agents are often additive.

Combination Therapy

Available combinations include diuretics/β-blockers, diuretics/ACE inhibitors, diuretics/ARBs, and ACE inhibitors/CCBs. Using a combination improves efficacy in certain patient groups who may not usually respond to certain agents. For example, in black patients, an ACE inhibitor or an ARB may be ineffective or only partially effective as monotherapy, or a small dose of a diuretic (12.5 mg/day) may not always lower BP to goal levels; a combination of small doses of each of these different classes of drugs is usually highly effective. The available antihypertensive medication combinations are listed in **Table 15**.**6**.

Figure 15.**1** outlines the approach that we follow in most cases of stage 1 and, in some cases, stage 2 hypertension. As noted previously, in patients at high risk (ie, diabetes, two or more other risk factors, etc), specific medications should be started along with lifestyle changes rather than waiting for several months to see what effect nonpharmacologic therapy might have. This is true even in patients with stage 1 or grade 1 hypertension (BP 140-160/90-100 mm Hg). In patients with stage 2 hypertension with BP of >160/100 mm Hg, especially those with evidence of LVH, we will start combination therapy without attempting a period of monotherapy, ie, using a combination of β-blocker/diuretic, ACE inhibitor/diuretic, or ARB/diuretic. The JNC 7 has recommended this approach as treatment. This type of treatment may appear to contradict the rule that we have all been taught: not to initiate therapy with several medications. One could argue that if the patient responds, you will not know

15

TABLE 15.6 — COMBINATION ANTIHYPERTENSIVE MEDICATIONS

Generic Name	Trade Name	Available Dosages (mg)
ACE Inhibitors and Diuretics		
Benazepril/hydrochlorothiazide	Lotensin HCT	5/6.25, 10/12.5, 20/12.5, 20/25
Captopril/hydrochlorothiazide	Captozide*	25/15, 25/25, 50/15, 50/25
Enalapril/hydrochlorothiazide	Vaseretic	5/12.5, 10/25
Fosinopril/hydrochlorothiazide	Monopril HCT	10/12.5, 20/12.5
Lisinopril/hydrochlorothiazide	Prinzide; Zestoretic	10/12.5, 20/12.5, 20/25
Moexipril/hydrochlorothiazide	Uniretic	7.5/12.5, 15/12.5, 15/25
Quinapril/hydrochlorothiazde	Accuretic	10/12.5. 20/12.5, 20/25
Angiotensin II Receptor Blockers and Diuretics		
Candesartan/hydrochlorothiazide	Atacand HCT	16/12.5, 32/12.5
Eprosartan/hydrochlorothiazide	Teveten HCT	600/12.5, 600/25
Irbesartan/hydrochlorothiazide	Avalide	150/12.5, 300/12.5
Losartan/hydrochlorothiazide	Hyzaar	50/12.5, 100/25

Olmesartan/hydrochlorothiazide	Benicar HCT	20/12.5, 40/12.5, 40/25
Telmisartan/hydrochlorothiazide	Micardis HCT	40/12.5, 80/12.5
Valsartan/hydrochlorothiazide	Diovan HCT	80/12.5, 160/12.5, 160/25
β-Adrenergic Blockers and Diuretics		
Atenolol/chlorthalidone	Tenoretic	50/25, 100/25
Bisoprolol/hydrochlorothiazide	Ziac*	2.5/6.25, 5/6.25, 10/6.25
Metoprolol/hydrochlorothiazide	Lopressor HCT	50/25, 100/25, 100/50
Nadolol/bendroflumethiazide	Corzide	40/5, 80/5
Propranolol (XR)/hydrochlorothiazide	Inderide LA	80/50
Timolol/hydrochlorothiazide	Timolide	10/25
Calcium Channel Blockers and ACE Inhibitors		
Amlodipine/benazepril	Lotrel	2.5/10, 5/10, 5/20, 10/20
Felodipine/enalapril	Lexxel	2.5/5, 5/5
Trandolapril/verapamil XR	Tarka	2/180, 1/240, 2/240, 4/240

Continued

15

Generic Name	Trade Name	Available Dosages (mg)
Other Combinations		
Amiloride/hydrochlorothiazide	Moduretic	5/50
Clonidine/chlorthalidone	Clorpres	0.1/15, 0.2/15, 0.3/15
Methyldopa/hydrochlorothiazide	Aldoril	250/15, 250/25, 500/30, 500/50
Prazosin/polythiazide	Minizide	1/0.5, 2/0.5, 5/0.5
Reserpine/chlorthalidone	Diupres	250/0.125, 500/0.125
Reserpine/thiaizde	Hydropres	25/0.125, 50/0.125
Spironolactone/hydrochlorothiazide	Aldactazide	25/25, 50/50
Triamterene/hydrochlorothiazide	Dyazide, Maxzide	37.5/25, 75/50

Abbreviations: ACE, angiotensin-converting enzyme; XR, extended release

* Approved for initial therapy.

which drug was effective. This may be true, but does it make a difference if BP is normalized and medication is well tolerated?

To reemphasize, when small doses of two drugs are used instead of large doses of one drug:

- The response rate to therapy is increased from about 40% to 50% to ≥70% to 80%
- Racial and age differences in response to different medications are mostly eliminated
- Frequency of office visits may be reduced
- BP is lowered more quickly
- Side effects are not increased (or are actually minimized)
- Cost is not increased to a great extent and may actually be less in some cases.

If BP remains normal after 1 year, one of the agents could be reduced or withdrawn. We find this approach to therapy practical in the "real world" and recent recommendations suggest a similar approach.

Combination Medications as Initial Therapy

A combination of a cardioselective β-blocker and a diuretic has been approved and is available as initial therapy for hypertension: bisoprolol/hydrochlorothiazide. This medication (Ziac) contains a small dose of the diuretic (6.25 mg) and is available with different doses of the β-blocker (2.5, 5, and 10 mg).

Approval of the drug followed the demonstration that although the low-dose individual components of the combination were only effective in about 20% to 25% of subjects, the combination lowered BP to goal levels in more than two thirds of patients. Importantly, because of the small doses of each component, side effects were similar to those with placebo. Placebo-controlled studies have demonstrated that this combi-

15

nation is as effective or more effective in lowering BP than an ACE inhibitor (enalapril) or a CCB (amlodipine). In addition, side effects were less frequent with the β-blocker/diuretic combination than with the other medications. Other β-blocker/diuretic combinations such as Corzide, Tenoretic, and Lopressor HCT are also effective with a high response rate.

An ACE inhibitor/thiazide diuretic combination (Captozide) has also been approved for initial therapy. Duration of action is prolonged and response rates increased when a diuretic is combined with the ACE inhibitor. While other combinations of ACE inhibitors/ diuretics have not been approved by the Food and Drug Administration (FDA) as initial therapy, these combinations are also acceptable and effective as initial therapy (**Table 15.6**). As repeatedly emphasized, an ARB/diuretic combination is effective with relatively minor side effects.

Some investigators advocate an approach that does not include a diuretic: eg, an ACE inhibitor, if ineffective, add a CCB, or start with a β-blocker and if this is ineffective, add a dihydropyridine CCB. As noted, when an ACE inhibitor is combined with a CCB (ie, benazepril/amlodipine), response rates are greater than with either agent alone and side effects, especially peripheral edema, are less. These combinations that do not contain a diuretic may be effective, but in our experience, a higher percentage of patients will respond if the treatment regimen includes a diuretic.

Newer Medications

Several newer medications and different uses for older drugs are curently under study. Some of these include:

- Agents that act centrally to decrease sympathetic nerve activity and which may also affect some of the metabolic abnormalities often noted in hypertensive individuals. Rilmenidine is an example of this group of agents that bind selectively to I_1 Imidazoline receptors.

- Drugs that are more selective aldosterone antagonists and that may modify CV risk. Eplerenone is an example of these compounds, which appear to be effective in cases of heart failure and are being extensively studied for their use in hypertension. Eplerenone has recently been approved by the FDA for use in hypertension and is awaiting approval for the treatment of heart failure. Data indicate that side effects, such as gynecomastia, are infrequent with eplerenone compared with spironolactone, an aldosterone antagonist that has been available for many years, and that BP lowering is equivalent to ACE inhibitors. This compound should prove to be of value in the treatment of hard-to-treat hypertensives as well as in many other patients with hypertension, especially when combined with a thiazide diuretic. Studies with eplerenone in combination with an ACE inhibitor or an ARB are also under way. There is still some concern regarding hyperkalemia when the agents are combined.

- Agents that combine several components (an ACE inhibitor plus a neutral endopeptidase inhibitor that prevents the breakdown of vasodilator substances). Omapatrilat is an example of this new class of agents, the vasopeptidase inhibitors. These drugs:
  - Block the conversion of angiotensin I to angiotensin II and its effect on vasoconstriction and sodium retention (ACE inhibitor action); and
  - Block the effects of neutral endopeptidase, which degrades vasodilatory natiuretic pep-

15

tides. This latter action potentiates the effect of natiuretic substances and increases the antihypertensive effects of ACE inhibitors. Although this is an effective BP-lowering agent and presents some theoretic advantages, studies indicate some potentially serious side effects. This medication has not been approved by the FDA.

Several other newer medications that block the effects of endothelin, a potent vasoconstrictor, as well as renin and vasopressor inhibitors, are being studied.

16 Management of the Patient With Resistant Hypertension

While there are some cases of resistant hypertension, ie, patients who do not achieve goal blood pressure (BP) levels on at least three different medications (one of which is a diuretic), these are relatively rare. There are several types of resistant hypertensives, two of which are illustrated in the following case studies.

Case #1

The first case illustrates the need for persistence on the part of the physician to continue to add, change, or uptitrate medications in order to achieve goal BP, especially in a high-risk patient.

A 62-year-old man with BP ranging between 170-180/100-110 mm Hg was first seen approximately 9 months ago. He had been referred to the clinic because of persistently high BP and a family history of diabetes. Findings included:

- Evidence of left ventricular hypertrophy (LVH) on electrocardiogram
- 1-plus proteinuria indicating an excretion of at least 300 mg/day protein
- Essentially normal physical examination with no evidence of abdominal bruit
- Fasting blood glucose level of 132 mg/dL
- Serum creatinine 1.7 mg/dL
- Other chemistries within normal limits.

This patient was diagnosed as a stage 2 hypertensive with diabetic nephropathy and had other evidence

241

of target-organ involvement (LVH); he was a high-risk patient. Based upon recent recommendations of the American Diabetes Association and other national committees and specific studies in diabetics with nephropathy, the patient was placed on a combination of an angiotensin II receptor blocker (ARB) and a thiazide; in this case, losartan 50 mg/hydrochlorothiazide 12.5 mg (Hyzaar) (this was an appropriate first step).

The patient was seen again within 2 to 3 weeks. Serum creatinine now was 2.6 mg/dL, BP had decreased to 155/95 mm Hg, and proteinuria was still present. The medication was doubled to losartan 100 mg/hydrochlorothiazide 25 mg, and the patient was again seen in 2 weeks. (It is not unusual to see an initial increase in serum creatinine levels as BP is lowered; however, if the creatinine levels continue to rise, this might provide a clue to the presence of renovascular hypertension.)

Several weeks later, BP was still 150-155/95 mm Hg. Serum creatinine levels had stabilized at 2.4 mg/dL and 1-plus proteinuria persisted. (Numerous studies have demonstrated that patients with diabetes and evidence of renal disease can be resistant to therapy and may require as many as three or more medications to bring BP under control.) In this instance, the physician who saw him decided that the patient was on maximum treatment and continued with the same therapy despite the fact that goal BP had not been achieved. Shortly after the third visit, the patient went on the internet and accessed the Seventh Joint National Committee (JNC 7) Report on Prevention, Detection, Evaluation, and Treatment of High Blood Pressure, which clearly stated that goal BP in a patient with hypertension and any type of kidney disease or diabetes was <130/80-85 mm Hg, so he sought help from a hypertension specialist in another facility.

Upon the initial visit to the hypertension specialists, it was determined that BP was still about 150-155/

95 mm Hg, with a creatinine level of 2.4 mg/dL. The ARB/diuretic combination was continued and a calcium channel blocker (CCB) was added (amlodipine 5 mg/day). It was only after several more visits that the BP decreased to <140/90 mm Hg. Over the ensuing several months, the serum creatinine level decreased to 1.5 mg/dL with a disappearance of proteinuria.

Long-term follow-up in this type of patient indicates that prognosis is reasonably good. Renal disease progression can be slowed if BP is kept as close to 120/80 mm Hg as possible (certainly at levels <130/80-85 mm Hg). This patient illustrates a case of resistant hypertension, but resistant only to the point where pharmacologic therapy was not adequate until a third class of medication was added.

Case #2

The second case is more common—an elderly person with isolated systolic hypertension (ISH) who experiences some symptoms as BP is lowered. A 2-stage or 2-step approach is often necessary to achieve a BP level as close to goal as possible consistent with noninterference with enjoyment of life.

A 76-year-old black female had persistent BP levels of 170-180/80 mm Hg. The physician initially ignored this BP level since the patient was asymptomatic and her physical examination was essentially negative. An electrocardiogram showed minimal voltage changes characteristic of LVH. Urinalysis was negative and blood glucose level was normal, with a serum creatinine level of 1.2 mg/dL.

16

When the physician was out of town and the patient saw a colleague, she was informed that her BP was elevated and that recent data have shown that even in patients >75 years of age, lowering BP is useful in reducing the occurrence of stroke and heart failure. The patient was appropriately started on a small dose of a diuretic (hydrochlorothiazide 12.5 mg), consistent with recommendations of most national committees on the treatment of ISH. She was seen in 2 to 3 months (an appropriate approach to treatment since management did not have to be as carefully monitored as in someone with more severe hypertension or renal disease). After several visits, however, BP levels remained $\geq 160/80-85$ mm Hg and, although there was some decrease in systolic blood pressure (SBP), which might conceivably reduce the risk for stroke or heart failure, the new physician decided that an alteration of strategy was needed to lower the SBP if possible. The diuretic was increased to 25 mg/day and a small dose of a β-blocker (metoprolol 25 mg) was added to treatment (this is considered appropriate therapy, although a small dose of an ACE inhibitor, ARB, or CCB would have also been appropriate).

BP did decrease slightly, but the patient began to experience some fatigue and dizziness on standing. Dosages were increased; there was an increase in symptoms. Finally, the patient decided to stop all medications. BP returned to previous levels; on the second attempt several months later, SBP was lowered to 150-160 mm Hg with the use of a diuretic and an ACE inhibitor and kept at this level for several months before increasing medication. (It is not unusual for elderly patients to experience some symptoms as SBP is reduced from 170-180 mm Hg to lower levels. It is prudent to suspend an increase in therapy at least for a few weeks while baroreceptors reset: a 2-stage or 2-step approach to therapy.) With this approach and the use of only 12.5 mg hydrochlorothiazide and a small dose of an ACE inhibitor (ramipril 5 mg), the patient's SBP decreased to 140-150 mm Hg. Although this is not considered ideal, it was considered by the physician to be the best that could be done without changing the quality of life for this patient. (There are many such elderly patients

244

in whom, despite multiple changes of medication, BP cannot be reduced below the goal BP of 140 mm Hg without some problems. However, all efforts should be made to reduce BP to goal levels, if at all possible.) Occasionally, SBP will decrease over time without any further change in therapy.

Summary

As noted elsewhere, many of the patients who are not treated to goal BP are patients with elevated SBP—and unlike the treatment of this patient, medications are not titrated or changed despite continued high SBP levels.

Although these two cases illustrate more frequent causes of resistance to therapy, there are obviously other reasons for nonresponsiveness to therapy, including:

- Lack of patient adherence to therapy (ie, forgetting to take medication, dropping out of therapy, cost of care, etc)
- Secondary causes of hypertension (ie, renovascular disease, pheochromocytoma, primary aldosteronism)
- Chronic use of nasal drops or medications for allergies that contain vasoconstrictor substances
- Use of steroids.

16

17 Results of Therapy

Remarkable progress has been made in the management of hypertension since the 1950s. **Figures 17.1** and **17.2** outline the percent decline in age-adjusted mortality since 1972 when the National High Blood Pressure Program was initiated. It should be noted that while noncardiovascular diseases have decreased by only about 12%, death from stroke has decreased by >60% in both sexes and in both black and white individuals from 148/100,000 in 1970 to 61/100,000 in 2000. Not all of this decrease, of course, can be attributed to better control of hypertension, since people are smoking less, exercising more, increasingly aware of cholesterol levels, etc. But since hypertension is present in almost 75% of patients with stroke, a good part of the decline can probably be attributed to better management of hypertension. In addition, a >50% decrease in coronary heart disease (CHD) deaths has also been noted; again, in both sexes and in blacks and whites from 483/100,000 in 1970 to 258/100,000 in 2000.

Obviously, as discussed above, there are factors other than better management of hypertension that may account for this dramatic response:

- People are:
  - Smoking less
  - Exercising more
  - Controlling other risk factors (ie, hyperlipidemia, taking aspirin)
- The advent of bypass surgery
- Better management of acute coronary events.

The specific results of hypertension treatment are dramatic. There have been >25 major trials since the

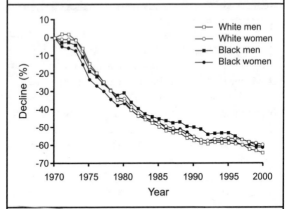

FIGURE 17.1 — PERCENT DECLINE IN AGE-ADJUSTED MORTALITY RATES FOR STROKE BY GENDER AND RACE: UNITED STATES, 1970-2000

Death rates are age-adjusted to the 2000 US census population.

Source: Prepared by T. Thom, National Heart, Lung, and Blood Institute from Vital Statistics of the United States, National Center for Health Statistics.

1970s. When the first 17 of these placebo or control studies are analyzed in **Figure 4.1**, we see that there has been a:

- 38% highly statistically significant decrease in stroke morbidity and mortality
- 16% highly statistically significant reduction in CHD events
- 21% statistically significant decrease in vascular mortality in treated compared with control or placebo subjects
- 52% decrease in the *occurrence* of congestive heart failure (CHF)
- 35% decrease in the *occurrence* of left ventricular hypertrophy (LVH) in treated compared with control patients.

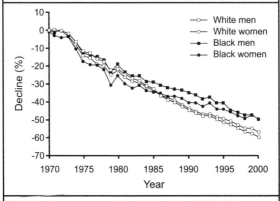

FIGURE 17.2 — PERCENT DECLINE IN AGE-ADJUSTED MORTALITY RATES FOR CORONARY HEART DISEASE BY GENDER AND RACE: UNITED STATES, 1970-2000

Death rates are age-adjusted to the 2000 US census population.

Source: Prepared by T. Thom, National Heart, Lung, and Blood Institute from Vital Statistics of the United States, National Center for Health Statistics.

These trials used diuretics and β-blockers primarily, with several other drugs, such as centrally acting or vasodilator drugs (α-methyldopa, reserpine, or hydralazine) being added if no response was noted. None of these trials used angiotensin-converting enzyme (ACE) inhibitors, angiotensin II receptor blockers (ARBs), or calcium channel blockers (CCBs) because they were not available when the studies were launched. However, it is clear that effective lowering of blood pressure (BP) with drugs available even 15 to 30 years ago produced excellent results. Results are even more dramatic when considering the fact that ≥25% of the subjects in these trials did not even achieve a goal diastolic blood pressure (DBP) <90 mm Hg.

17

However, in addition to the hard end points of stroke, stroke deaths, myocardial infarction (MI), and MI deaths, there are other benefits that have accrued from the lowering of BP. **Table 17.1** summarizes all of the trials from which data were available relating to progression of disease; these were placebo or controlled trials. In the placebo or control groups, 1493 of 13,342 patients progressed to more severe disease with systolic blood pressure (SBP) >200 to 210 mm Hg and DBP >110 to 120 mm Hg compared with only 95 of 13,389 patients in the treated group. This benefit of therapy represents a "soft end point," but it indicates that early treatment of hypertension prevents progression.

Table 17.2 presents details of the effects of treatment on the prevention of LVH in treated compared with control subjects. A highly significant decrease of 35% in the number of patients who developed LVH in the treated compared with the control group was noted. While most physicians recognize that LVH is often decreased by lowering BP, many of them are not aware that this major risk factor for sudden death and heart failure can actually be prevented.

It is of interest to note that several long-term follow-up studies indicate that hypertensive patients with LVH who experience regression of LVH following BP lowering live longer with fewer morbid events than those who do not lower BP levels.

Table 17.3 presents details from the clinical trials demonstrating the dramatic 52% reduction in the occurrence of CHF in treated compared with control subjects in the clinical trials. These are impressive data, suggesting the importance of the management of hypertension as a measure for the *prevention* of heart failure.

CHF remains an increasingly common reason for hospitalization, especially in individuals >60 years of age. Newer therapies, ie, the use of ACE inhibitors,

TABLE 17.1 — EFFECT OF TREATMENT ON PREVENTING PROGRESSION FROM LESS-SEVERE TO MORE-SEVERE HYPERTENSION*: FINDINGS FROM MAJOR CLINICAL TRIALS

Study (Range for Mild-Moderate Hypertension—mm Hg)	Placebo Group		Active Treatment	
	No.	Progressed to More Severe	No.	Progressed to More Severe
Total	13,342	1493	13,389	95

* Diastolic blood pressure > 110 mm Hg, systolic blood pressure >200-210 mm Hg.

From: *J Am Coll Cardiol.* 1996;27:1214.

TABLE 17.2 — LEFT VENTRICULAR HYPERTROPHY REPORTED IN RANDOMIZED TRIALS OF BLOOD PRESSURE LOWERING

	Active Treatment		Control Treatment	
	LVH	No. Randomized	LVH[†]	No. Randomized
Total: All Trials	140*	6150	215	6078

* Significant reduction of 35% in the occurrence of left ventricular hypertrophy (LVH) in treated compared with control subjects.

From: *J Am Coll Cardiol.* 1996;27:1214.

TABLE 17.3 — CONGESTIVE HEART FAILURE REPORTED IN RANDOMIZED TRIALS OF BLOOD PRESSURE LOWERING*

	Active Treatment		Control Treatment	
	CHF	No. Randomized	CHF	No. Randomized
Total: 12 Trials	112	6914	240	6923

Relative risk 0.48—Treatment:control; 95% confidence interval—0.38, 0.59

* *A reduction of 52% in the occurrence of congestive heart failure (CHF) in treated compared with control subjects was noted in these controlled, randomized hypertension treatment trials.*

From: *J Am Coll Cardiol.* 1996;27:1214.

ARBs, α_1–β-blockers such as carvedilol, and some β-blockers such as bisoprolol and metoprolol, in addition to diuretics and digitalis, have helped to prevent *recurrence* of CHF and its symptoms. Far more important, however, from both the patient's point of view and the economics of health care, is the prevention of the occurrence of heart failure in the first place.

Hypertension, as noted, has been identified as a major factor in the cause of CHF. It is probable that if more hypertensive patients were treated more effectively, the occurrence of CHF would decrease still further. Although the total number of CHF cases in the United States has actually increased over the past few years, a good part of the increase is closely related to the fact that people are living longer and not dying from acute MI or serious arrhythmias as often as before (ie, there has been an increase in survival from ischemic heart disease events).

The Newer Comparative Trials

The Hypertension Optimal Treatment (HOT), the Captopril Prevention Project (CAPPP), the Swedish Trial in Old Persons with Hypertension 2 (STOP-Hypertension-2), Nordic Diltiazem (NORDIL), International Nifedipine Gastrointestinal Therapeutic System Study Intervention as a Goal for Hypertension Therapy (INSIGHT) trial, United Kingdom Prospective Diabetes Study (UKPDS), the Antihypertensive and Lipid-Lowering Treatment to Prevent Heart Attack Trial (ALLHAT), and the Australian National Blood Pressure (ANBP 2) trial were comparative studies and were not placebo controlled. Therefore, results cannot be combined with findings from controlled trials. However, when event rates from some of these studies are compared with estimated rates from epidemiologic studies, they are consistently lower, suggesting ongoing and increasing benefits of treatment. It is doubtful, for ethical reasons, that there will be any additional placebo-controlled trials planned in the future in hypertensive patients, but comparative treatment studies are important and provide information regarding the relative benefits of different approaches to therapy, especially in specific population groups.

The treatment data in patients with renal disease with and without diabetes have repeatedly demonstrated that lowering BP with an ACE inhibitor–based or ARB-based regimen (usually including a diuretic) will slow down progression of renal disease. Although the total number of patients with end-stage renal disease (ESRD), as monitored by dialysis statistics, has increased in the United States, the reasons also include the fact that people are not dying from cardiovascular (CV) events at earlier ages, diabetics are living longer, and people are being accepted for dialysis at much older ages than they were 15 to 20 years ago.

Results of Therapy in the Elderly

Many large trials over the past 15 to 20 years have shown that morbidity and mortality from cerebrovascular and CV events can be reduced significantly in elderly hypertensives, including patients >75 years of age, by lowering BP (**Table 17.4**). Treatment of systolic and diastolic hypertension, as well as isolated systolic hypertension (ISH), in the elderly has decreased heart failure, stroke, and CHD events. One of the trials, the Systolic Hypertension in the Elderly Program (SHEP) (**Figure 17.3**), employed small doses of a diuretic with a β-blocker added, if necessary, and demonstrated:

- A marked 37% reduction in strokes
- 25% reduction in transient ischemic attacks
- 30% reduction in MIs
- 54% reduction in the occurrence of CHF when compared with placebo.

17

TABLE 17.4 — EFFECTS OF THERAPY IN OLDER HYPERTENSIVE PATIENTS

	CLINICAL TRIAL NAME							
	Australian	EWPHE	C & W	STOP	MRC	SHEP	HDFP	Syst Eur
Number of patients	582	840	884	1,627	4,396	4,736	2,374	4,695
Age range (years)	60-69	> 60	60-79	70-84	65-74	60 ≥ 80	60-69	> 60
Mean blood pressure at entry (mm Hg)	165/101	182/101	197/100	195/102	185/91	170/77	170/101	174/86
Percent Reduction of Events in Treated Compared to Controls								
Stroke	33	36	42*	47*	25*	33*	44*	42*
CAD	18	20	+ 0.03	13†	19	27*	15*	30
CHF	—	22	32	51≈	—	55*	—	29
All CVD	31	29*	24*	40*	17*	32*	16*	31*

Abbreviations: C & W, Coope and Warrender; CAD, coronary artery disease; CHF, congestive heart failure; CVD, cerebrovascular disease; EWPHE, European Working Party on High Blood Pressure in the Elderly; HDFP, Hypertension Detection and Follow-up Program; MRC, Medical Research Council Study; SHEP, Systolic Hypertension in the Elderly Program; STOP, Swedish Trial in Older Patients With Hypertension; Syst Eur, Systolic Hypertension in Europe.

* Statistically significant.
† Myocardial infarction only; sudden deaths decreased from 13 to 4.

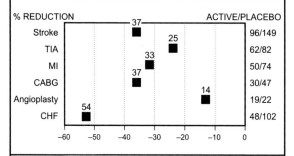

FIGURE 17.3 — SHEP: NONFATAL EVENTS

% REDUCTION		ACTIVE/PLACEBO
Stroke	37	96/149
TIA	25	62/82
MI	33	50/74
CABG	37	30/47
Angioplasty	14	19/22
CHF	54	48/102

Abbreviations: CABG, coronary artery bypass graft; CHF, congestive heart failure; MI, myocardial infarction; TIA, transient ischemic attack.

Percent reduction in nonfatal events in the Systolic Hypertension in the Elderly Program (SHEP).

JAMA. 1991;265:3255-3264.

Benefit was noted in diabetic subjects and in patients with hyperlipidemia. A review of the diuretic- or β-blocker–based trial data in elderly hypertensives notes that diuretics will reduce BP to goal levels in a higher percentage of subjects than β-blockers. In addition, although the β-blocker–based trials demonstrated a reduction in stroke and CHF in treated compared with control subjects, the reduction in CHD events was not significant. In contrast, diuretic-based therapy in the elderly has reduced not only stroke and CHF, but also CHD events. The Sixth Joint National Committee on Prevention, Detection, Evaluation, and Treatment of High Blood Pressure (JNC 6) *recommendations included the use of diuretics or β-blockers and diuretics as initial therapy in the elderly with systolic/diastolic hypertension.* This was an appropriate recommendation based on data available in 1997. The JNC 7 report suggests a thiazide diuretic as initial therapy in most cases but that a thiazide combination with another

17

agent may be necessary in many patients to achieve goal BP.

It should be reemphasized, however, that the use of β-blockers post-MI has resulted in a significant reduction in CHD morbidity and mortality in both low-risk and high-risk patients (ie, those without too many additional complicating factors or those with other risk factors [poor cardiac function]). Many elderly hypertensive patients have some evidence of ischemic heart disease.

As noted in a study of subjects primarily with ISH (Systolic Hypertension in Europe [Syst Eur]), nitrendipine, a moderately long-acting dihydropyridine CCB (not available in the United States), was given as initial therapy with an ACE inhibitor or diuretic added, if necessary. Fatal and nonfatal strokes were reduced (**Table 17.4**). Therapy with the CCB plus other agents (enalapril and/or a diuretic) decreased overall CV events to a greater degree than monotherapy. Based on the Syst Eur data, a long-acting dihydropyridine may be considered for monotherapy in elderly patients with ISH if a diuretic is contraindicated or ineffective.

In contrast to this recommendation, the World Health Organization–International Society of Hypertension (WHO-ISH) and the European Societies of Hypertension and Cardiology reports recommend a medication from any of the six classes of antihypertensive drugs (ie, diuretics, β-blockers, ACE inhibitors, ARBs, CCBs, or α-blockers) as acceptable initial treatment. As noted in the Swedish Trial in Older Patients With Hypertension 2 (STOP-Hypertension-2) study, overall mortality and morbidity were similar in the diuretic/β-blocker group when compared with an ACE inhibitor/CCB–treated group but the ACE inhibitor group experienced fewer episodes of CHF and MI than the CCB group. In ALLHAT, which primarily was a study in the elderly (mean age 67 years), CHD events were similar among the three groups. There were fewer episodes of heart failure with a thiazide diuretic than with CCBs and fewer overall CV events than with an ACE inhibitor (secondary outcomes).

In the SCOPE trial (mean age 76 years), a regimen based on the use of an ARB (candesartan) significantly reduced nonfatal stroke when compared with a regimen that did not include the ARB. Based on all of the accumulated data, it is probably fair to conclude that a thiazide should be the drug of choice for initial therapy in most elderly patients whether they have systolic and diastolic hypertension or ISH. Although CCBs, ACE inhibitors, and ARBs lower BP and are reasonably well tolerated in the elderly population, these medications should probably be considered as alternative or add-on therapy or for use in special situations. For further comments about this recommendation, see Chapter 4, *Drug Treatment of Hypertension*: *General Information.*

In our experience, older patients respond well to combinations of small doses of a diuretic/β-blocker, ACE inhibitor or ARB/diuretic combination, or a CCB with a diuretic, and this may represent a reasonable approach to therapy. There are, however, no long-term morbidity and mortality data available at this time for these specific therapies. Occasionally, the use of an ACE inhibitor/diuretic or ARB/diuretic once daily in addition to a β-blocker/diuretic once daily will result in excellent BP control in patients who may not previously have been controlled. Usually, few side effects result from these regimens.

A reasonable approach is to stabilize and not increase therapy if a patient notes fatigue or dizziness with an initial decrease in SBP, for example, 180 mm Hg to 150-160 mm Hg. After a 3- to 6-week period of time after baroreceptors have been reset, a further attempt can be made to reduce BP still further by increasing medication (a 2-stage approach to treatment).

17

Goal SBP may not always be achievable in elderly patients (**Figure 17.4**).

It may not always be possible to achieve an exact BP target, especially in elderly patients, but the lowest possible BP (<140/90 mm Hg) without producing side effects should actually be the goal of therapy. In the elderly, numerous studies (ALLHAT, CONVINCE, etc) have reported that DBP goals of <90 mm Hg can be achieved in 90% or more of patients. In some elderly subjects with ISH, only a 20-25 mm Hg reduction in SBP from levels of 170 to 175 mm Hg to about 150 mm Hg might be achievable, but even this degree of reduction has been shown to reduce CV events.

Treatment of Hypertension in the Very Old (>80 Years of Age)

One might question why anyone would wish to treat a functioning man or woman of 80-plus years with BP of ≥160-180/80-85 mm Hg. Does benefit exceed the possible cost or annoyance of therapy? Occasionally, sodium restriction will be effective in decreasing BP to some extent, but in most cases, medication will be necessary to decrease SBP even by 15-20 mm Hg.

The results of therapy in this age group are of interest. Results in >1800 patients >80 years of age who have been treated in various controlled trials are noted in **Table 17.5** (data for the ALLHAT in the >80-year-old group have not been included since this was a comparative drug trial).

While longevity may not be increased by treatment in these very elderly hypertensives, two major disabling conditions (stroke and heart failure) appear to be significantly decreased. Treatment is worthwhile. These results have been achieved with only a modest BP reduction of 10-15/5-6 mm Hg (compared with control subjects). Better results might be anticipated with even better BP control.

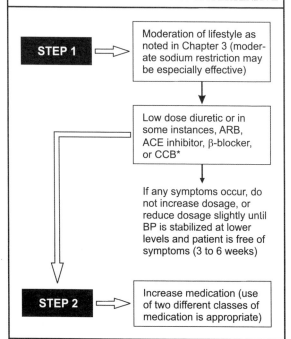

FIGURE 17.4 — APPROACH TO THE MANAGEMENT OF THE ELDERLY HYPERTENSIVE

STEP 1 ⟹ Moderation of lifestyle as noted in Chapter 3 (moderate sodium restriction may be especially effective)

↓

Low dose diuretic or in some instances, ARB, ACE inhibitor, β-blocker, or CCB*

↓

If any symptoms occur, do not increase dosage, or reduce dosage slightly until BP is stabilized at lower levels and patient is free of symptoms (3 to 6 weeks)

STEP 2 ⟹ Increase medication (use of two different classes of medication is appropriate)

Abbreviations: ACE, angiotensin-converting enzyme; ARB, angiotensin II receptor blocker; CCB, calcium channel blocker.

* If initial blood pressure is >180 mm Hg or patient has evidence of renal disease, coronary heart disease, or diabetes, the use of combination therapy for initial treatment represents a reasonable approach.

17

TABLE 17.5 — RESULTS OF ANTIHYPERTENSIVE DRUG THERAPY IN PATIENTS >80 YEARS OF AGE*

• Significant reduction of:
  – >35% in strokes (mostly nonfatal)
  – >35% in heart failure
  – >20% in cardiovascular events
• Nonsignificant reduction of about 20% in major coronary events
• Nonsignificant increase of about 10% to 15% in total mortality

* Based on results in >1800 patients.

Treatment need not be expensive or interfere with the enjoyment of life if medication is chosen carefully and dosages are titrated slowly and in stages.

The New Trial Data and Treatment Decisions

How then should the practitioner use these new data for treatment decisions? Should the JNC 7 recommendations for initial therapy be accepted? Based on data from several trials like the United Kingdom Prospective Diabetes Study (UKPDS), a conclusion could be drawn that BP lowering by any means (usually with multiple drugs) is more important in most cases than the specific therapy used. This is the conclusion that the WHO-ISH and European committees reached when they suggested that any of the available effective medications (ie, diuretics, β-blockers, ACE inhibitors, ARBs, CCBs, or α-blockers) could be used as initial therapy. However, α-blockers appear to have been eliminated for this choice by the results of the Antihypertensive and Lipid-Lowering Treatment to Prevent Heart Attack Trial (ALLHAT).

Choices then among the five other classes may relate to tolerability and cost. But in some cases, there does appear to be a difference between classes of drugs, such as:

- Some data suggest that ACE inhibitors reduce CV events more than CCBs in diabetics and in the elderly; although ALLHAT, in which the mean age was 67 years and that included 14,000 diabetic patients, did not report a difference in CHD outcome between an ACE inhibitor and a CCB
- Diuretics may reduce CHF more than CCBs
- ACE inhibitors, β-blockers, or ARBs appear to reduce progression of renal disease to a greater degree than a dihydropyridine CCB (**Table 17.6**)
- One trial suggests that a nondihydropyridine CCB may reduce stroke to a greater degree than a diuretic.
- An ARB reduces death from CV disease, all-cause mortality, and heart failure more than a β-blocker–treatment regimen in diabetic hypertensive patients with LVH.

One review of long-term trials had suggested about a 20% greater incidence of CHF and MI events when a CCB is used as baseline therapy compared with the use of other agents, but in the ALLHAT, there was no difference in fatal and nonfatal MIs among patients treated with a CCB, an ACE inhibitor, or a diuretic.

Specific recommendations that take these data into account are outlined in Chapter 15, *Approach to Treatment: Combination Therapy*.

Final Comments

17

In managing hypertension, it is up to the individual physician to decide on a specific medication as initial or subsequent therapy. The JNC 7, WHO-ISH, and European reports all advance the concept of titrating

TABLE 17.6 — COMPARATIVE MORBIDITY/MORTALITY OUTCOME DATA WITH ANTIHYPERTENSIVE MEDICATIONS

CCBs Compared With Diuretics
- MIDAS Trial: fewer CV events in diuretic group compared with short-acting dihydropyridine CCB (isradipine)
- VHAS: No difference in outcome, nondihydropyridine CCB (verapamil) and diuretic
- INSIGHT: No *overall* difference in CV events with long-acting dihydropyridine (nifedipine) and diuretic, but fewer fatal MIs and episodes of CHF with diuretic
- NORDIL: Significantly fewer strokes with nondihydropyridine CCB (diltiazem) but trend toward more MIs and CHF than with diuretic/β-blocker
- ALLHAT: No difference in fatal or nonfatal MIs; more CHF than with a diuretic

CCBs Compared With ACE Inhibitor
- ABCD and FACET: Fewer vascular events in type 2 diabetics in ACE inhibitor group compared with long-acting dihydropyridine group (small number of patients)
- STOP-Hypertension-2: Fewer MIs and less CHF with ACE inhibitor compared with a dihydropyridine CCB
- AASK: Progression of renal disease less with ACE inhibitor than with a dihydropyridine CCB in black patients with proteinuria
- ALLHAT: No difference in fatal or nonfatal CHD events between a CCB and an ACE inhibitor
- INVEST: CCBs (+ ACE inhibitor) compared with β-blocker (+ thiazide) in patients with CHD; no difference in CV events; less new-onset diabetes in CCB group

ACE Inhibitors Compared With β-Blockers
- UKPDS: No difference in outcome in type 2 diabetics if tight blood pressure control achieved
- CAPPP: No difference in overall events; fewer strokes in β-blocker group; better outcome in diabetics with ACE inhibitor (poor randomization)

ACE Inhibitors/CCBs Compared With Diuretic/β-Blocker
- STOP-Hypertension-2: No overall difference in outcome between older and newer drugs

ACE Inhibitors Compared With Diuretics
- ANBP 2: Marginally better outcome with ACE inhibitor; only in men

ARBs Compared With Dihydropyridine CCB
- IDNT: Less progression of renal disease with ARB than with CCB in patients with type 2 diabetic nephropathy

ARBs Compared With β-Blocker
- LIFE study: in hypertensives with LVH, fewer strokes, new-onset diabetes, and overall CV events; in diabetics, fewer deaths from CV disease, less heart failure, and lower all-cause mortality with an ARB

Diuretics Compared With β-Blocker
- MRC Trial in the Elderly: Better blood pressure control and more favorable outcome with diuretics

Alpha-Blocker Compared With Diuretic
- ALLHAT: Better blood pressure control and fewer CV events, especially heart failure, with diuretic compared with doxazosin

Abbreviations: AASK, African American Study of Kidney Disease; ABCD, Appropriate Blood Pressure in Control in Diabetes; ACE, angiotensin-converting enzyme; ALLHAT, Antihypertensive and Lipid-Lowering Treatment to Prevent Heart Attack Trial; ANBP 2, Australian National Blood Pressure; ARB, angiotensin II receptor blocker; CAPPP, Captopril Prevention Project; CCB, calcium channel blocker; CHF, congestive heart failure; CV, cardiovascular; FACET, Fosinopril Versus Amlodipine Cardiovascular Events Trial; IDNT, Irbesartan Diabetic Nephropathy Trial; INSIGHT, International Nifedipine Gastrointestinal Therapeutic System Study: Intervention as a Goal in Hypertension Treatment; INVEST, International Verapamil SR/Trandolapril Study (INVEST); LIFE, Losartan Intervention for Endpoint Reduction in Hypertension; MI, myocardial infarction; MIDAS, Multicenter Isradipine Diuretic Atherosclerosis Study; MRC, Medical Research Council [study]; NORDIL, Nordic Diltiazem [trial]; STOP-Hypertension-2, Swedish Trial in Older Patients With Hypertension 2; UKPDS, United Kingdom Prospective Diabetes Study; VHAS, Verapamil in Hypertension Atherosclerosis Study.

17

with one, or in many cases, two or even three medications plus lifestyle interventions until goal BP is reached.

As noted repeatedly in this book, there is a large body of evidence from carefully conducted long-term clinical trials that effective and long-term management of hypertension with the agents currently available will reduce not only so-called "hard end points" such as stroke and stroke deaths, MIs, and CHD death, but also many of the other complications that were previously noted in untreated subjects.

In addition, there are also increasing amounts of data to indicate benefit of BP lowering in preventing renal insufficiency, especially in diabetics. There is some concern that patients who are not treated early enough or in whom BP is not lowered to <135-140/85-90 mm Hg will progress to renal insufficiency. Lowering BP to <130-135/80-85 mm Hg is especially important in diabetic patients to prevent progression to renal failure. It is speculated that delayed or inadequate therapy is a major reason for the number of hypertensive patients with ESRD who require dialysis, especially in black patients and in diabetics.

Further progress must be made in increasing the number of patients with hypertension who are controlled. A recent survey that only about 55% to 60% of patients with hypertension were being treated and that only about 35% of all hypertensives are being controlled at levels <140/90 mm Hg (**Table 17.7**). Recent studies (ALLHAT, CONVINCE, etc) have demonstrated that >60% of patients can be controlled if a specific protocol is followed and physicians are motivated to achieve goal BP of <140/90 mm Hg in most cases and <130/80-85 mm Hg in patients with diabetes or renal disease. Some physicians may still not be aware of the major benefits of therapy and may not be implementing therapy early enough or pursuing it vigorously enough to achieve good results, especially in older patients and in patients with ISH.

TABLE 17.7 — TRENDS IN AWARENESS, TREATMENT, AND CONTROL OF HIGH BLOOD PRESSURE IN ADULTS WITH HYPERTENSION AGE 18 TO 74 YEARS

Percent	National Health and Nutrition Examination Surveys, Weighted %			
	II 1976-1980	III (Phase 1) 1988-1991	III (Phase 2) 1991-1994	1999-2000
Awareness	51	73	68	70
Treated*	31	55	53	59
Controlled*	10	29	27	34

* Systolic blood pressure of <140 mm Hg and diastolic blood pressure of <90 mm Hg.

The JNC 7 Report. *JAMA*. 2003;289:2562.

17

There is some concern that the trend in benefits of lowering BP (ie, stroke reduction) is slowing down and efforts must be made to increase the number of patients under effective treatment.

A clear message should be sent that BP lowering to a goal of <140/90 mm Hg or even lower in patients with diabetes or renal disease, if at all possible, has been shown to be beneficial at any age. Concerns about reducing BP too much and possibly increasing the risk of an MI have largely been put to rest, in our opinion, by the results of the Hypertension Optimal Treatment (HOT) study in which DBP was reduced to <80-85 mm Hg in subjects with ischemic heart disease without ill effects, and the Systolic Hypertension in the Elderly Program (SHEP) study in which average DBP was reduced to <70 mm Hg with a decrease, not an increase, in CV events in patients with abnormal baseline electrocardiograms.

With the advent of newer agents that may act more physiologically or may act on other risk factors, we may be able to improve the results of treatment. But it should be emphasized that available medications are effective in a large majority of patients if titrated properly. We have the tools to do a better job. The important point to remember is that if we are going to achieve results as good as or better than those achieved in the clinical trials, careful attention must be paid to:

- Keeping the regimen as simple as possible
- Keeping expense of treatment at a reasonable level
- Setting a goal of BP levels of at least <140/90 mm Hg and adhering to this goal as closely as possible.

This may not always be easy to achieve but in the majority of patients, it is possible. Patient adherence to therapy and achievements of goal BP will improve if more attention is paid to these principles.

18 Selected Readings

Diagnosis

2003 European Society of Hypertension-European Society of Cardiology guidelines for the management of arterial hypertension. *J Hypertens.* 2003;21:1011-1053.

Chobanian AV, Bakris GL, Black HR, et al, and the National High Blood Pressure Education Program Coordinating Committee. The Seventh Report of the Joint National Committee on Prevention, Detection, Evaluation, and Treatment of High Blood Pressure. The JNC 7 Report. *JAMA.* 2003;289:2560-2572.

Gifford R, Moser M. Initial workup of the hypertensive patient. In: Izzo JL, Black HR, eds. *Hypertension Primer: The Essentials of High Blood Pressure.* Philadelphia, Pa: Lippincott, Williams and Wilkins; 2003:325-328.

Joint National Committee on Prevention, Detection, Evaluation, and Treatment of High Blood Pressure. The Fifth Report of the Joint National Committee on Detection, Evaluation, and Treatment of High Blood Pressure (JNC-V). *Arch Intern Med.* 1993;153:154-183.

Joint National Committee on Prevention, Detection, Evaluation, and Treatment of High Blood Pressure. The Sixth Report of the Joint National Committee on Detection, Evaluation, and Treatment of High Blood Pressure (JNC-VI). *Arch Intern Med.* 1997;157: 2413-2446.

Julius S, Mejia A, Jones K, et al. "White coat" versus "sustained" borderline hypertension in Tecumseh, Michigan. *Hypertension.* 1990;16:617-623.

Levy D, Anderson KM, Savage DD, Kannel WB, Christiansen JC, Catelli WP. Echocardiographically detected left ventricular hypertrophy: prevalence and risk factors. The Framingham Heart Study. *Ann Intern Med.* 1988;108:7-13.

Pickering TG, Devereux RB. Ambulatory monitoring of blood pressure as a predictor of cardiovascular risk. *Am Heart J.* 1987;114: 925-928.

Lifestyle/Nonpharmacologic Interventions

Appel LJ, Moore TJ, Obarzanek E, et al. A clinical trial of the effects of dietary patterns on blood pressure. DASH Collaborative Research Group. *N Engl J Med.* 1997;336:1117-1124.

Beilin LJ. Alcohol, hypertension and cardiovascular disease. *J Hypertens.* 1995;13:939-942. Editorial.

Cushman WC, Cutler JA, Hanna E, et al. Prevention and Treatment of Hypertension Study (PATHS): effects of an alcohol treatment program on blood pressure. *Arch Intern Med.* 1998;158:1197-1207.

Cutler JA, Follmann D, Allender PS. Randomized trials of sodium reduction: an overview. *Am J Clin Nutr.* 1997;65(suppl 2):643S-651S.

Hypertension Prevention Trial Research Group. The Hypertension Prevention Trial: three-year effects of dietary changes on blood pressure. *Arch Intern Med.* 1990;150:153-162.

Langford HG, Davis BR, Blaufox MD, et al. Effect of drug and diet treatment of mild hypertension on diastolic blood pressure. The TAIM Research Group. *Hypertension.* 1991;17:210-217.

Linas SL. The role of potassium in the pathogenesis and treatment of hypertension. *Kidney Int.* 1991;39:771-786.

Stamler R, Stamler J, Gosch FC, et al. Primary prevention of hypertension by nutritional-hygienic means. Final report of a randomized, controlled trial. *JAMA.* 1989;262:1801-1807.

Stamler R, Stamler J, Grimm R, et al. Nutritional therapy for high blood pressure. Final report of a four-year randomized controlled trial—the Hypertension Control Program. *JAMA.* 1987;257:1484-1491.

Trials of Hypertension Prevention Collaborative Research Group. The effects of nonpharmacologic interventions on blood pressure of persons with high normal levels. Results of the Trials of Hypertension Prevention, Phase I. *JAMA.* 1992;267:1213-1220.

Whelton PK, Appel LJ, Espeland MA, et al. Sodium reduction and weight loss in the treatment of hypertension in older persons: a randomized controlled trial of nonpharmacologic interventions in the elderly (TONE). TONE Collaborative Research Group. *JAMA*. 1998;279:839-846.

World Hypertension League. Alcohol and hypertension—implications for management. A consensus statement by the World Hypertension League. *J Hum Hypertens*. 1991;5:227-232.

Pharmacologic Therapy

2003 European Society of Hypertension-European Society of Cardiology guidelines for the management of arterial hypertension. *J Hypertens*. 2003;21:1011-1053.

Chobanian AV, Bakris GL, Black HR, et al, and the National High Blood Pressure Education Program Coordinating Committee. The Seventh Report of the Joint National Committee on Prevention, Detection, Evaluation, and Treatment of High Blood Pressure. The JNC 7 Report. *JAMA*. 2003;289:2560-2572.

Borhani NO, Mercuri M, Borhani PA, et al. Final outcome results of the Multicenter Isradapine Diuretic Atherosclerosis Study (MIDAS). A randomized controlled trial. *JAMA*. 1996;276:785-791.

Dahlor B, Devereux RB, Kjeldsen SE, et al. Cardiovascular morbidity and mortality in the Losartan Intervention For Endpoint reduction in hypertension study (LIFE): a randomised trial against atenolol. *Lancet*. 2002;359:995-1003.

Eisen SA, Miller DK, Woodward RS, Spitznagel E, Przybeck TR. The effect of prescribed daily dose frequency on patient medication compliance. *Arch Intern Med*. 1990;150:1881-1884.

Gifford RW Jr. Management of hypertensive crises. *JAMA*. 1991;266:829-835.

Gurwitz JH, Bohn RL, Glynn RJ, Monane M, Mogun H, Avorn J. Antihypertensive drug therapy and the initiation of treatment for diabetes mellitus. *Ann Intern Med*. 1993;118:273-278.

18

Hypertension Detection and Follow-up Program Cooperative Group. Five-year findings of the Hypertension Detection and Follow-up Program (HDFP), 1. Reduction in mortality of persons with high blood pressure, including mild hypertension. *JAMA.* 1979;242:2562-2571.

Joint National Committee on Prevention, Detection, Evaluation, and Treatment of High Blood Pressure. The Fifth Report of the Joint National Committee on Detection, Evaluation, and Treatment of High Blood Pressure (JNC-V). *Arch Intern Med.* 1993;153:154-183.

Joint National Committee on Prevention, Detection, Evaluation, and Treatment of High Blood Pressure. The Sixth Report of the Joint National Committee on Detection, Evaluation, and Treatment of High Blood Pressure (JNC-VI). *Arch Intern Med.* 1997;157: 2413-2446.

Materson BJ, Reda DJ, Cushman WC, et al. Single-drug therapy for hypertension in men. A comparison of six antihypertensive agents with placebo. The Department of Veterans Affairs Cooperative Study Group on Antihypertensive Agents. *N Engl J Med.* 1993;328:914-921.

Materson BJ, Reda DJ, Williams D. Lessons from combination therapy in Veterans Affairs Studies. Department of Veterans Affairs Cooperative Study Group on antihypertensive agents. *Am J Hypertens.* 1996;9:187S-191S.

Moser M. Antihypertensive medications: relative efficacy and adverse reactions. *J Hypertens.* 1990;8(suppl):S9-S16.

Moser M. The cost of treating hypertension: can we keep it under control without compromising the level of care? *Am J Hypertens.* 1998;11:120S-127S, discussion 135S-137S.

Moser M. Current hypertension management: separating fact from fiction. *Cleve Clin J Med.* 1993;60:27-37.

Moser M. Diuretics revisited—again. *J Clin Hypertens.* 2001; 3:136-138.

Moser M. National recommendations for the pharmacological treatment of hypertension: should they be revised? *Arch Intern Med.* 1999;159:1403-1406.

Moser M. Why are physicians not prescribing diuretics more frequently in the management of hypertension? *JAMA*. 1998;279: 1813-1816.

Moser M, Ross H. The treatment of hypertension in diabetic patients. *Diabetes Care*. 1993;16:542-547.

Multiple Risk Factor Intervention Trial Research Group. Mortality rates after 10.5 years for participants in the Multiple Risk Factor Intervention Trial. Findings related to a prior hypotheses of the trial. *JAMA*. 1990;263:1795-1801.

National High Blood Pressure Education Program Working Group on high blood pressure in pregnancy. Working Group Report on high blood pressure in pregnancy. *Am J Obstet Gynecol*. 1990; 163:1691-1712.

Neaton JD, Grimm RH Jr, Prineas RJ, et al. Treatment of Mild Hypertension Study (TOMHS). Final results. Treatment of Mild Hypertension Study Group. *JAMA*. 1993;270:713-724.

Papademetriou V, Burris JF, Notargiacomo A, Fletcher RD, Freis ED. Thiazide therapy is not a cause of arrhythmia in patients with systemic hypertension. *Arch Intern Med*. 1988;148:1272-1276.

Pollare T, Lithell H, Berne C. A comparison of the effects of hydrochlorothiazide and captopril on glucose and lipid metabolism in patients with hypertension. *N Engl J Med*. 1989;321:868-873.

PROGRESS Collaborative Group. Randomised trial of a perindopril-based blood-pressure–lowering regimen among 6105 individuals with previous stroke or transient ischaemic attack. *Lancet*. 2001;358:1033-1041.

Tarazi RC, Dustan HP, Frohlich ED. Long-term thiazide therapy in essential hypertension. Evidence for persistent alteration in plasma volume and renin activity. *Circulation*. 1970;41:709-717.

World Health Organization–International Society of Hypertension. 1999 World Health Organization–International Society of Hypertension guidelines for the management of hypertension. Guidelines Subcommittee. *J Hypertens*. 1999;17: 151-183.

18

■ Results of Therapy

The ALLHAT Officers and Coordinators for the ALLHAT Collaborative Research Group. Major cardiovascular events in hypertensive patients randomized to doxazosin vs chlorthalidone: the Antihypertensive and Lipid-Lowering Treatment to Prevent Heart Attack Trial (ALLHAT). *JAMA.* 2000;283:1967-1975.

Black HR, Elliott WJ, Grandits G, et al. Principal results of the Controlled Onset Verapamil Investigation of Cardiovascular End Points (CONVINCE) trial. *JAMA.* 2003;289:2073-2082.

Brown MJ, Palmer CR, Cataigne A, et al, for the INSIGHT Study Group. Morbidity and mortality in patients randomised to double-blind treatment with a long-acting calcium channel blocker or diuretic in the International Nifedipine GITS Study: Intervention as a Goal in Hypertension Treatment (INSIGHT). *Lancet.* 2000;356: 366-372.

Burt VL, Culter JA, Higgins M, et al. Trends in the prevalence, awareness, treatment, and control of hypertension in the adult US population. Data from the health examination surveys, 1960 to 1991. *Hypertension.* 1995;26:60-69.

Cushman WC, Ford CE, Cutler JA, et al. Success and predictors of blood pressure control in diverse North American settings: the Antihypertensive and Lipid-Lowering Treatment to Prevent Heart Attack Trial (ALLHAT). *J Clin Hypertens.* 2002;4:393-405.

Dahlof B, Devereux RB, Kjeldsen SE, et al. Cardiovascular morbidity and mortality in the Losartan Intervention For Endpoint reduction in hypertension study (LIFE): a randomised trial against atenolol. *Lancet.* 2002;359:995-1003.

Hansson L, Lindholm LH, Niskanen L, et al. Effect of angiotensin-converting-enzyme inhibition compared with conventional therapy on cardiovascular morbidity and mortality in hypertension; the Captopril Prevention Project (CAPP) randomised trial. *Lancet.* 1999;353:611-616.

Hansson L, Hedner T, Lund-Johansen P, et al, for the NORDIL Study Group. Randomised trial of effects of calcium antagonists compared with diuretics and β-blockers on cardiovascular morbidity and mortality in hypertension: the Nordic Diltiazem (NORDIL) study. *Lancet.* 2000;356:359-365.

Hansson L, Zanchetti A, Carruthers SG, et al. Effects of intensive blood-pressure lowering and low-dose aspirin in patients with hypertension: principal results of the Hypertension Optimal Treatment (HOT) randomised trial. HOT Study Group. *Lancet.* 1998;351:1755-1762.

Heart Outcome Prevention Evaluation (HOPE) Study Investigators. Effects of ramipril on cardiovascular and microvascular outcomes in people with diabetes mellitus: results of the HOPE study and the MICRO-HOPE substudy. *Lancet.* 2000;255:253-259.

Hebert PR, Moser M, Mayer J, Glynn RJ, Hennekens CH. Recent evidence on drug therapy of mild to moderate hypertension and decreased risk of coronary heart disease. *Arch Intern Med.* 1993;153:578-581.

Major outcomes in high-risk hypertensive patients randomized to angiotensin-converting enzyme inhibitor or calcium channel blocker vs diuretic: The Antihypertensive and Lipid-Lowering Treatment to Prevent Heart Attack Trial (ALLHAT). *JAMA.* 2002;288:2981-2997.

McMurray JJ, Ostergren J, Swedberg K, et al, for the CHARM Investigators and Committees. Effects of candesartan in patients with chronic heart failure and reduced left-ventricular systolic function taking angiotensin-converting-enzyme inhibitors: the CHARM-Added trial. *Lancet.* 2003;362:767-771.

Moser M, Hebert P, Hennekens CH. An overview of the meta-analyses of the hypertension treatment trials. *Arch Intern Med.* 1991;151:1277-1279.

Moser M, Hebert PR. Prevention of disease progression, left ventricular hypertrophy and congestive heart failure in the hypertension treatment trials. *J Am Coll Cardiol.* 1996;27:1214-1218.

Moser M. Angiotensin converting enzyme inhibitors, angiotensin II receptor antagonists and calcium channel blocking agents: a review of potential benefits and possible adverse reactions. *J Am Coll Cardiol.* 1997;29:1414-1421.

Moser M. Treating hypertension: calcium channel blockers, diuretics, β-blockers, ACE inhibitors. Is there a difference? *J Clin Hyper.* 2000;2:301-304.

18

Neal B, MacMahon S, Chapman N; Blood Pressure Lowering Treatment Trialists' Collaboration. Effects of ACE inhibitors, calcium antagonists, and other blood-pressure-lowering drugs: results of prospectively designed overviews of randomised trials. Blood Pressure Lowering Treatment Trialists' Collaboration. *Lancet.* 2000;356:1955-1964.

PROGRESS Collaborative Group. Randomised trial of a perindopril-based blood-pressure-lowering regimen among 6105 individuals with previous stroke or transient ischaemic attack. *Lancet.* 2001;358:1033-1041.

Wright JT Jr, Bakris G, Greene T, et al, for the African American Study of Kidney Disease and Hypertension Study Group. Effect of blood pressure lowering and antihypertensive drug class on progression of hypertensive kidney disease: results from the AASK trial. *JAMA.* 2002;288:2421-2431.

Yusuf S, Peto R, Lewis J, Collins R, Sleight P. Beta blockade during and after myocardial infarction: an overview of the randomized trials. *Prog Cardiovasc Dis.* 1985;27:335-371.

■ Treatment of the Diabetic Patient

Brenner BM, Cooper ME, de Zeeuw D, et al. Effects of losartan on renal and cardiovascular outcomes in patients with type 2 diabetes and nephropathy. *N Engl J Med.* 2001;345:861-869.

Estacio RO, Jeffers BW, Hiatt WR, Biggerstaff SL, Gifford N, Schrier RW. The effect of nisoldipine as compared with enalapril on cardiovascular outcomes in patients with non-insulin-dependent diabetes and hypertension. *N Engl J Med.* 1998;338:645-652.

Lewis EJ, Hunsicker LG, Clarke WR, et al. Renoprotective effect of the angiotensin-receptor antagonist irbesartan in patients with nephropathy due to type 2 diabetes. *N Engl J Med.* 2001;345:851-860.

Lindholm LH, Ibsen H, Bahlof B, et al. Cardiovascular morbidity and mortality in patients with diabetes in the Losartan Intervention For Endpoint reduction in hypertension study (LIFE): a randomised trial against atenolol. *Lancet.* 2002;359:1004-1010.

Parving HH, Lehnert H, Brochner-Mortensen J, Gomis R, Andersen S, Arner P. The effect of irbesartan on the development of diabetic nephropathy in patients with type 2 diabetes. *N Engl J Med.* 2001;345:870-878.

Tatti P, Pahor M, Byington RP, et al. Outcome results of the fosinopril versus amlodipine cardiovascular events randomized trial (FACET) in patients with hypertension and NIDDM. *Diabetes Care*. 1998;21:597-603.

United Kingdom Prospective Diabetes Study Group. Efficacy of atenolol and captopril in reducing risk of macrovascular and microvascular complications in type 2 diabetes: UKPDS 39. *BMJ*. 1998;317:713-720.

United Kingdom Prospective Diabetes Study Group. Tight blood pressure control and risk of macrovascular and microvascular complications in type 2 diabetes: UKPDS 38. *BMJ*. 1998;317:703-713.

■ Treatment of the Elderly

Curb JD, Pressel SL, Cutler JA, et al. Effect of diuretic-based antihypertensive treatment on cardiovascular disease risk in older diabetic patients with isolated systolic hypertension. Systolic Hypertension in the Elderly Program Cooperative Research Group. *JAMA*. 1996;276:1886-1892.

Dahlof B, Lundholm L, Hansson L, Schersten B, Ekbom T, Wester P. Morbidity and mortality in the Swedish Trial in Older Patients with Hypertension (STOP-Hypertension). *Lancet*. 1991;338:1281-1285.

Hansson L, Lindholm LH, Ekborn T, et al. Randomised trial of old and new antihypertensive drugs in elderly patients: cardiovascular mortality and morbidity in the Swedish Trial in Old Patients With Hypertension-2 Study. *Lancet*. 1999;354:1751-1756.

Lithell H, Hansson L, Skoog I, et al. The Study on Cognition and Prognosis in the Elderly (SCOPE): principal results of a randomized double-blind intervention trial. *J Hypertens*. 2003;21:875-886.

MRC Working Party. Medical Research Council trial of treatment of hypertension in older adults: principal results. *BMJ*. 1992;304: 405-412.

Moser M. Approach to the treatment of hypertenison in the octogenarian. *J Clin Hypertens*. 2000;2:366-368.

Rosei EA, Dal Palu C, Leonetti G, Magnani B, Pessina A, Zanchetti A. Clinical results of the verapamil in hypertension and atherosclerosis study. VHAS Investigators. *J Hypertens*. 1997;15:1337-1344.

18

SHEP Cooperative Research Group. Prevention of stroke by anti-hypertensive drug treatment in older persons with isolated systolic hypertension. Final results of the Systolic Hypertension in the Elderly Program (SHEP). *JAMA*. 1991;265:3255-3264.

Staesson JA, Fagard R, Thijs L, et al. Randomised double-blind comparison of placebo and active treatment for older patients with isolated systolic hypertension. The Systolic Hypertension-Europe (Syst Eur) Trial Investigators. *Lancet*. 1997;350:757-764.

Staesson L, Thijs L, Fagard R, et al. Calcium channel blockade and cardiovascular prognosis in the European trial in isolated systolic hypertension. *Hypertension*. 1998;32:410-416.

Wing LM, Reid CM, Ryan P, et al, for the Second Australian National Blood Pressure Study Group. A comparison of outcomes with angiotensin-converting—enzyme inhibitors and diuretics for hypertension in the elderly. *N Engl J Med*. 2003;348:583-592.

INDEX

19

19

281

19

19

286

19

288

19

19

19

294

19

19

19

19

19